An Account of Rural Medical Practice from the 18th century onwards

in

Long Buckby, Northamptonshire.

by

Dr. R. Graham Lilly, MB.BS., MRCGP

Retired
General Practitioner

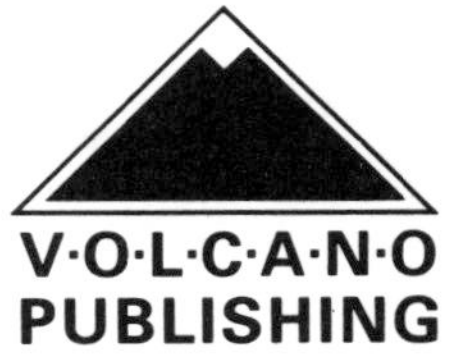

Volcano Publishing,
13 Little Lunnon,
Dunton Bassett,
Leics. LE17 5JR

© R. Graham Lilly 1993

Printed and bound in England.

Phototypeset in 10pt Times Roman.

This book is sold subject to the condition that
it shall not, by way of trade or otherwise, be lent,
re-sold, hired out, or otherwise circulated without
the publisher's prior, consent.

All rights reserved. No part of this publication may be
reproduced or transmitted in any form or by any means,
electronic or mechanical, including photography, recording or
any information storage or retrieval system, without permission
in writing from the publisher.

ISBN 1 870127 99 4

To

Cynthia Churchouse

In thanks for her help,
friendship and support
in my early years, and

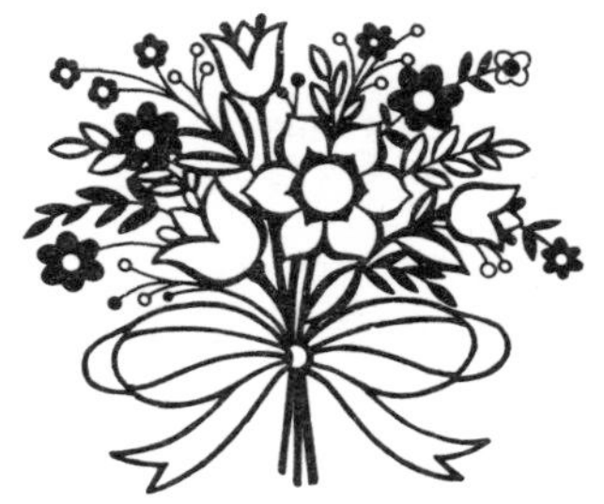

To

Marie, my wife

for her long, loyal support.

Acknowledgements

Mr. J.J.B. Atkinson; Mr. F.G. Buswell;

Miss I. Cousins (Central Reference Library, Northampton)

the late A.G. Cox, JP; Mr. M.J.W. Churchouse; Mr. P.R. Davis;

Mr. K.H. Grace-Dutton; Mr. R.L. Greenall; Mr. D.B. Hughes;

Mr. P.I. King, Former County Archivist
and the present staff of the Northamptonshire Record Office;

Dr. S. Mattingly; Mrs. J.M. Raybould;

Dr. N.D. Richards
(Head, Dept. of Social Studies, Trent Polytechnic, Nottingham);

Mrs. George Thompson;

Wellcome Institute for the History of Medicine including former Library Assistant Heather Walkden, and present Library Assistant Judith Barker;

Mr. W.R. Green; and last but by no means least,
the late Victor A. Hatley for his kindness and advice.

I wish to thank the Automobile Association for permission to reproduce and photocopy the map opposite to the introduction.

The map on page 84 is reproduced from the 1988 Ordnance Survey 1:50,000 Northampton and Milton Keynes map, Sheet No. 152, with permission of the Controller of Her Majesty's Stationery Office.

© Crown Copyright.

The practice map on page 11 is reproduced by kind permission of Mrs. J.M. Raybould.

Thanks to Mr. Peter Clifton for permission to reproduce the photograph of Dr. Churchouse on page 34 and to Mrs. Margery Cox for the family photographs on pages 42-46 and of Holly House on pages 39 and 58.

Contents

List of Illustrations

Preface

This is in the nature of a brief apologia. My critics may complain that the chapters are insufficiently chronological: surely the 19th century follows the 18th? Similarly, at the end of the account, the earlier decades of the 20th century are followed by the second half of the present century.

If the table in Chapter 2 is not entirely clear, I can only plead that it is not to me either. The transition from the 18th to the 19th century was not cut and dried nor was it easy to fit in the numerous single, and limited-number, reference names in the earlier decades of the 19th century. Not only were the references scanty but the material in them was also.

I should like to pre-empt any criticsm of the middle section by stating that this is as much local history as medical. In fact I wrote the middle chapters first after I was enthralled by my reading of our fine series of old Parish Magazines and remarkly complete Minutes of Long Buckby Parish Council.

I simply felt that there was a good story – what better reason for writing? I researched the doctors later.

R. Graham Lilly

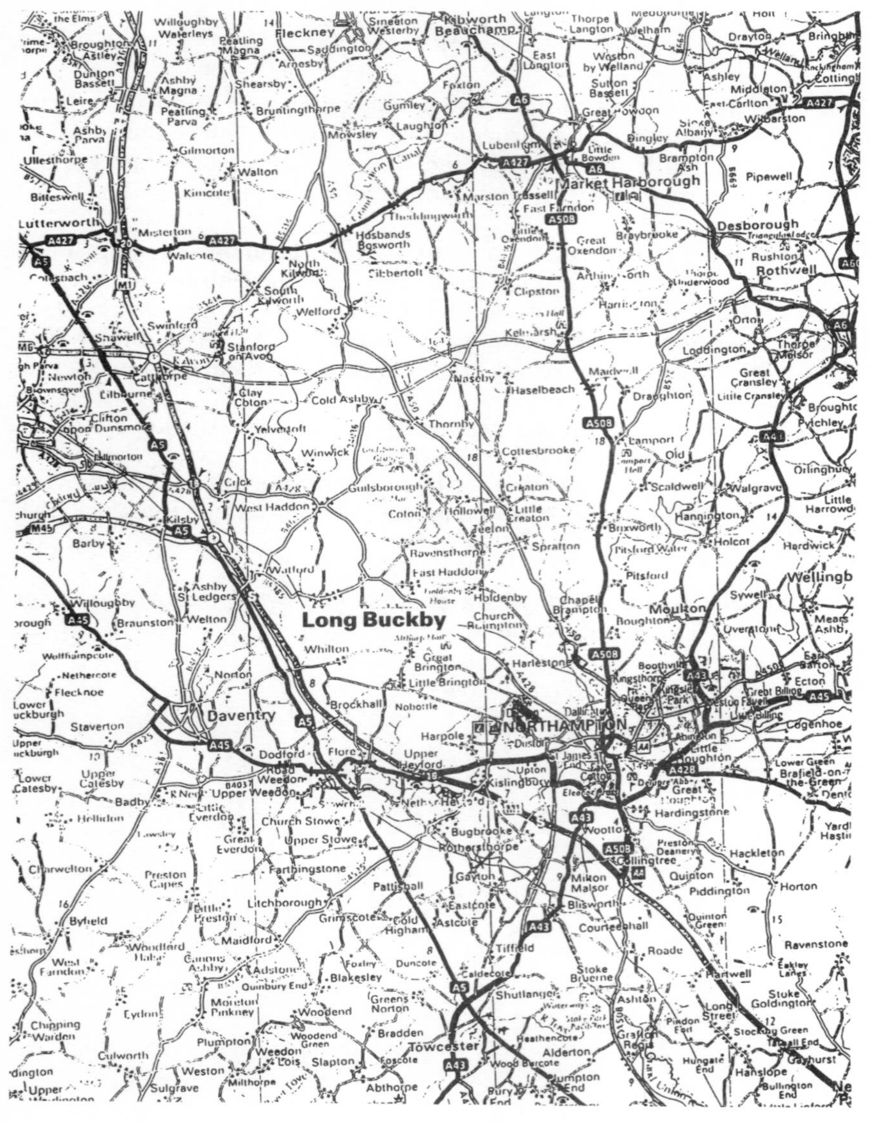

Long Buckby! – where is it?

Introduction

"...Let us go down to the Radical Village, I beg its pardon, the Town of Long Buckby." That is all very fine but where is it?

Long Buckby is 10 miles equidistant from the county town of Northampton and Rugby just over the Warwickshire border with Daventry 5 miles to the South West. It is near the famous Watford Gap used by Romans, 19th and 20th Century Civil engineers for their transport routes, and 2½ miles by road from the M1 Service Area of that ilk.

The prefix LONG was not apparently recorded until the 16th Century, but centuries before in the troubled times of Danish invasion, Buckebi was a settlement on the outskirts of Danelaw. It was, no doubt, a frontier observation post with the line between Danelaw and Wessex so near along the route of the Watling Street (the modern A5) at this point.

That it was an ancient settlement is shown by the steep-sided, sunken lanes (hollow ways) on the west slope of the high ground indicating medieval thoroughfares. This was the original village.

It went 'up market' with the construction of a ring motte castle with one bailey (perhaps originally two) built either in the first, or second half, of the 12th century. It was probably built by the de Quincy family, later Earls of Winchester, who by Henry II's reign held, and were to hold, the main manor of Long Buckby until 1264.

It increased still further in importance with the grant to Henry de Lacy, Earl of Lincoln, and his heirs, of a weekly market on Thursday at his manor of Buckeby, Co. Northampton. This Charter was created on November 2nd 1280. Two three-day fairs were also granted. While the market is no more the two fairs survive, although in different form; and were Long Buckby to stand on ceremony, it is entitled to be called a Chartered Market Town. The present village centre can thus be seen as a later, probably planned, addition to the earlier settlement to the west, set up in about 1280 by Henry de Lacy, Earl of Lincoln and Salisbury, when he was granted his Charter.

The development of the village and the character of the inhabitants over the centuries very largely resulted from one single fact; namely an Absentee Lord of the Manor. Long Buckby became an open village. Many villagers became independent of land and landowners; non-conformist preachers were eagerly listened to as were the later arguments of radical politicians. A good example of the contrast between an open village, such as Long Buckby with its strong non-conformist tradition, and the neighbouring estate village of East Haddon is well illustrated at the turn of the 19th Century. It occured during the long pastorate of Mr. Daniel Griffiths, Independent Minister for 30 years.

Mr. Griffiths used to 'lecture' once a month in a private house in East Haddon and so many people desired to hear him that the accommodation was soon insufficient and a chapel was built. This did not please the squire at that time and he gave notice to the farmers on his estate that if they continued to deal with, or employ, shopkeepers who attended dissenting services, they would be removed from their farms. Although legal help was sought, nothing effective could be done and the tradespeople concerned lost the custom of nearly all the farmers in the parish. In spite of these difficulties, the chapel was completed in 1811.[1]

When my account opens in the 18th Century, Long Buckby was prosperous. It was the centre of a woolcombing and worsted-weaving area – indeed towards the end of the wool boom there were names of 40 woolcombers and 21 weavers in the Long Buckby section of the 1777 Militia List. This, of course, included only men between the ages of 18 and 45.

The population was about 1,008 in 1720 and there was a gentle upward curve until 1801 when the figure was 1,500. Thereafter a steeper curve brought the population in 1821 to 1,843 (census). In the 19th Century a maximum of just over 2,500 was reached in 1881.

Non-conformity was strong. The Independent Chapel was founded in 1707 and the present building erected in 1771. During the Rev Richard Denny's long pastorate from 1763 there was an extraordinary revival in the congregation and, in the course of 2-3 years, about 40 members were added to the church.[2] During this period the Baptist Church was founded in 1759 and the present church on the Market Place was built in 1846. Later there were to be two other minor sects in the village.

Later there were to be two other minor sects in the village.

As the Vicar (C.A. Yate) said in 1872; "There is a General Baptist Chapel, A Particular Baptist Chapel and an independent Chapel. I should say fully ⅔ of the Parishioners are Dissenters. Of course prevalence of dissent is a hindrance to me. And there is also amongst the shoemakers a good deal of Infidelity", (non-believing and non-practice).

The wool industry declined rapidly around 1780 owing to industrial competition in Yorkshire. Thereafter there were great distress and hardship in the village until the burgeoning shoe industry, introduced from Daventry, becoming fully established in the 1840s.

So we come to 19th Century Radicalism. First there was Chartism. (1838-40, 1842-44, 1847-50). In 1843 a Chartist teetotal Working Men's Club was built (the old Junior School Canteen, now demolished). In 1842 the Rev A. Burdett, the Baptist Minister, addressed a Chartist meeting in the Market Place on Easter Monday. The Northern Star (Chartist newspaper) reported him as tracing the evils by which the country is borne down to their source, class legislation. So there we are. No one had a monopoly of politics.

The radical tradition continued by the invitation in 1881 of the Long Buckby Liberal and Radical Union to Mr. C. Bradlaugh, M.P. (the famous – for years – non-attesting M.P. for Northampton) to address an open-air meeting on 'Land Reform'. He was greeted at the entrance to the town with great enthusiasm. Note the use of the word town. The report used it and said he was met by the united brass bands! A procession was formed.

The radical torch continued to be carried, perhaps in a quieter and less militant way, by Long Buckby Women's Liberal Association, 1894 to 1913.

Finally a cause worthy of some inhabitants' protest, indignation and independence of mind was the 1902 Education Act. After this Act ratepayers' money was used to fund the Board Schools.

Passive Resistance.

First Prosecutions in Northamptionshire. Long Buckby Defendents

at Daventry. There were four summonses, all issued against residents at Long Buckby.
*The Rev. Thomas Ruston** (Independent Minister);
The Rev. A.C.G. Rendell (Baptist Minister);
Mr. James Eyre (shoe manufacturer);
and *Mr. Henry A. Underwood* (farmer).

All four were passive resisters – all had witheld sums from their rates. Rev. Ruston paid his sum in court after he had made his protest. As regards the other three, distraint against property was effected.

I think I have said enough to indicate what sort of place Long Buckby was – and is – and what the people were like.

Rerferences:

1. Ivory, Leslie S., Long Buckby Congregational Church 1707-1957. A Brief Historical Sketch, 1957.
2. Ibid, 1957.

* See *Polly and Alice* by Winifred Mary Ruston for further information about the village.

1. The Early Doctors

It is easy to say when scientific medicine began in Long Buckby; it began when medicine became scientific throughout the world. However, medicine being the youngest science, this was not until the late 1930s.

But when did the first doctors, or surgeons and apothecaries as we should call them in those days, practise? When did the first qualified pharmacist set up in place of shops selling human and veterinary – and especially horse – medicaments, old country remedies and old wives' cures along with other goods?

The 18th Century medical men turned out to be well documented; not at all the shadowy figures expected – merely names on Militia Lists, in Vestry Minutes and on Church Monuments.

The first reference in Northamptonshire Record Office to a surgeon/apothecary is Thomas West. Little is known of him. He bought a house (an Indenture Feoffment[1] for joint ownership of a Messuage Yard and Land costing £118-10s-0d dated 10th March 1729 is extant) and he made a will proved on 6th February 1740.

That he lived and died is important. And he was described as a surgeon in the Indenture Feoffment.

Hubert Floyer and Edward Swinfen – overlapping though not strictly contemporary – may be regarded as the founding fathers of medicine in Long Buckby. It was they who establised the traditions of two independent practices for nearly two centuries and of sons following fathers, not only into the profession, but often into the practice. Anthony Floyer (with a younger brother William in practice at Flore) followed his father. In Swinfen's case it was nepotism and he was succeeded by Samuel Harris. In the cases of Dix, Churchouse and Cox a son not only became a doctor but entered the practice. In the Dix, Cox, Watson and the writer's families, sons went in for medicine but did not practise in Long Buckby.

Who and what were the apothecaries and surgeons? For the 18th Century and the early part of the 19th Century the terms were synonomous. Men were not trained and examined – indeed they were not examined at all – in one or the other. Hubert Floyer was described as of Long Buckby, apothecary at his marriage to Mary Gundry of Long Buckby at All Saints, Northampton, in 1753. Apparently apothecaries were not excused Militia Service and Edward Swinfen was included under this heading in the Long Buckby Militia Lists of 1771, 1774 and 1777. Anthony Floyer was only on the 1777 list. Yet in 1802 Edward Swinfen was called Surgeon on his memorial tablet in the south aisle of Long Buckby Church.

Reference:

1 Feoffment – *Concise Oxford Dictionary* – n, a particular way of conveying freehold estate.

SACRED TO THE MEMORY OF
WILLIAM FLOYER, ESQ. SURGEON,
LATE OF THE PARISH OF FLOORE
IN THIS COUNTY,
IN THE YEAR OF HIS AGE.
HE PASSED A LONG AND ACTIVE LIFE USEFULLY
EMPLOYED IN THE DUTIES OF HIS PROFESSION
AND PRACTISED AT FLOORE FOR A PERIOD
OF FIFTY SEVEN YEARS.
THIS TABLET
IS ERECTED TO HIS MEMORY AS A TRIBUTE OF AFFECTION
BY HIS WIDOW
AND SURVIVING MEMBERS OF HIS FAMILY.
ANN FLOYER, WIFE OF THE ABOVE,
ALSO
HUBERT WILLIAM FLOYER, ELDER SON OF THE ABOVE
AGED 76 YEARS.

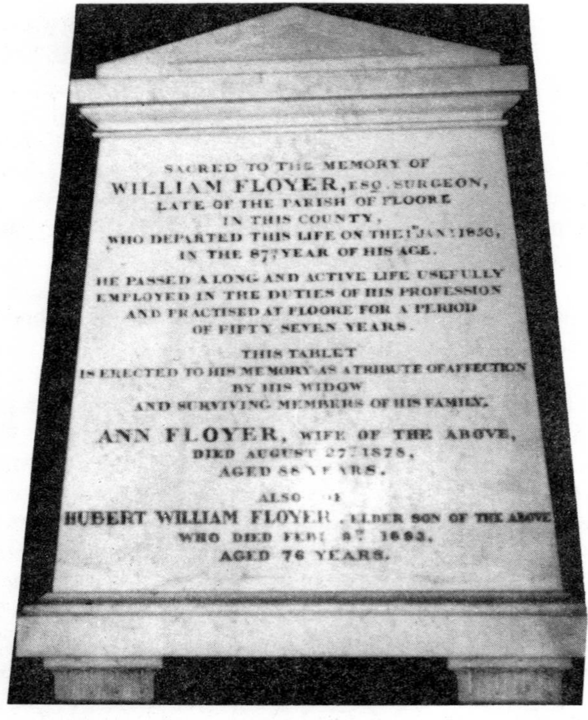

Memorial to Dr. Floyer in the church of St. Laurence, Long Buckby.

Samuel Swinfen Harris was referred to as a Surgeon in a newspaper account of 30th June 1810[1] and similarly in a conveyance dated 29th March 1837 recently perused and in private hands. Indeed it was only these last two chance findings that led me to know that there ever had been a surgeon called Harris in Long Buckby.

How were they trained? The one and only essential was apprenticeship for 5 to 7 years from the age of 15. For most aspirants this meant being bound to a provincial or country apothecary. Once certified by their Masters that they had diligently and satisfactorily concluded their apprenticeship they were qualified to set up in a vacancy or suitable location, join an establised practitioner in partnership – often their fathers – or work as a paid assistant.

Young men would always go to London and become apprenticed to the Barber-Surgeons' Company before 1745 and then to the Surgeons' Company after the Barbers and Surgeons separated. Newly created hospitals were opening in London where young men could learn more practical surgery in a month than in twelve months spent attending the Barber-Surgeons' lectures and demonstrations, few in number due to the cost, and hence the dearth, of obtaining hanged criminals' bodies for dissection. So surgical aspirants began to go direct to the surgeons of hospitals such as St. Thomas's and St. Bartholomew's rather than apprentice themselves to the Barber-Surgeons' Company. As many of the great hospitals which came into being in London in the early 18th Century often began as charitable dispensaries the surgical apprentices of the hospital surgeons could, presumably, learn the work of the apothecary as well. There were other ways you could learn your anatomy in London. Dr. William Hunter, elder brother of the great John Hunter, surgeon, pathologist, experimentor, was appointed the first Professor of Anatomy at the Royal Academy of Arts in 1768.[2,6] He obtained his cadavers illegally, although the R.A. overlooked this for the sake of good education, because it was not until 1832 that the Anatomy Act legalised dissection.[3] The European Magazine 1782, advertised the syllabus of courses of anatomy, physiology and surgery that could be undertaken by artists and anatomists alike.[4] Also advertised was a 'school for practical anatomy where students dissect with their own hands, and made for themselves many preparations'.[5]

References:
1. The late Harold Clifton's, *Long Buckby Archives:* "Mr. Harris, Surgeon, Long Buckby. 24th March 1810. On the night of the 24th last a fire broke out in the dwelling house of Mr. Harris, Surgeon, Long Buckby...nothing was insured...the loss is estimated at £1,500 (Northampton Mercury 30th June 1810)

The news took a long time to travel 11 miles. Perhaps fires were commonplace and hardly newsworthy but rumours of this enormous, uninsured loss gradually filtered across. *R.G.L.*

2. Art and Anatomy Revisited by Anne Darlington, *Journal of the Royal College of General Practitioners,* March 1987.
3. Ibid.
4. Ibid.
5. Ibid.
6. Two Centuries of Immunology etc. by Deborah Newton, *British Medical Journal, Volume 295,* 18th July 1987 — it seems John Hunter also had an Anatomy School attended by Edward Jenner who was also studying on the wards at St. George's Hospital.

So much for the metropolis. As the century wore on the same sort of thing was happening in the provinces. Voluntary hospitals were being founded – Northampton in 1743 – workhouses opened (not Unions; they were not built until after the Poor Law Amendment Act 1834) thus expanding the scope and opportunities for surgical apprenticeship.[1] So young surgical aspirants went direct to hospital surgeons. While they got good surgical teaching I am not sure how they obtained experience in apothecary work. How did those not gaining a surgical post in hospital acquire the apothecary's skills for a town or country practice? Maybe the physicians in hospital gave instruction in therapeutics and dispensing to cover this eventuality. Having said this I am sure young men could not be formally apprenticed to physicians, who were consultants, and that these (if any) semi-unofficial courses were not a 'back-stairs' and cheap way of becoming a physician. At this time the only way you could become a physician was to attend one of the only two English Universities of Oxford and Cambridge, where reliance on ancient authorities, which characterized such English 'medical' education as existed, was in stark contrast to the Scottish schools.[2] When Addenbrooke's Hospital was opened a contemporary comment was made that it would perhaps deflect criticism against university training, which was so theoretical that men went to European schools for further instruction.[3] Also when a charity sermon of 1777 was preached on behalf of the Salop Infirmary, it was noted that 'charitable hospitals' (are) now considered the best in physick (sic) and surgery' and that training there crowned the earlier part of medical instruction.[4]

In summary, therefore, at the outset some, probably most, of the would-be entrants to 'medicine' would only have aspired to 'G.P.' status and would have been content with apprenticeship to a 'G.P.' of the profession, though it must be pointed out that the term general practitioner was a much later innovation. As late as 1885 Kelly's Directory of Northamptonshire listed Arthur Cox as Surgeon and he was described in 1890 as Surgeon, Medical Officer and Public Vaccinator to No.4 District Daventry Union. The 1885 Kelly's Directory also listed Dix and Churchouse as Surgeons.

References:

1. Appendix 1. Woodward, J., To Do The Sick No Harm. A Study of the British Voluntary Hospital System to 1875, Routledge and Kegan Paul, London, Henly and Boston, 1974.

Ref.1 cont.

The Voluntary Hospitals of the eighteenth Century.

English Hospitals:

(a) LONDON	Date of opening
Westminster Hospital	1720
Guys Hospital	1724
St. George's Hospital	1733
London Hospital	1740
Middlesex Hospital	1745
In addition there were two general chartered institutions:	
St. Bartholomew's Hospital	1123 (refounded 1546)
St. Thomas's Hospital	1213 (refounded 1551)
(b) PROVINCES	
Winchester County	1736
Bristol Royal Infirmary	1737
York County Hospital	1740
Royal Devon and Exeter Hospital	1741
Bath General Hospital	1742
Northampton General Hospital	1743
Worcester Royal Infirmary	1746
Royal Salop Infirmary	1747
Liverpool Royal Infirmary	1749
Royal Victoria Infirmary, Newcastle-upon-Tyne	1751
Manchester Royal Infirmary	1752
Gloucester Royal Infirmary	1755
Chester Infirmary	1755
Addenbrooke's Hospital, Cambridge	1766
Salisbury County Hospital	1766
Staffordshire County Hospital	1766
Radcliffe Infirmary, Oxford	1770 etc...

Scottish Hospitals

Edinburgh Royal Infirmary	1729
Aberdeen Royal Infirmary	1742
Dumfries and Galloway Royal Infirmary	1778
Glasgow Royal Infirmary	1792
Dundee Royal Infirmary	1798

2. Waddy,F.F., A History of Northampton General Hospital, 1743 to 1948, *The Guildhall Press (Northampton) Ltd,* 1974, and Langford, A.W., The History of Hereford General Hospital, *Transactions of the Woolhope Naturalists' Field Club (Herefordshire),* 1959. See Appendix 1.
3. Quoted by Joan Lane in 'Medical Education in the Provinces in 18th Century England' from S. Hallifax. A sermon for the Governors of Addenbrooke's Hospital, Cambridge, 1771. (The History of Medical Education, Spring Conference, London 1987).
4. Quoted by Joan Lane, ibid, from W. Adams, Sermons and Tracts (Shrewsbury 1777).

Sir Luke Fildes's famous picture, now in the Tate Gallery, painted around 1878, was not called 'The General Practitioner', it was entitled 'The Doctor'.

In the late 18th Century it has been estimated that there were only about 3,100 qualified practitioners (according to Simmons's Medical Register for 1783) and probably up to twice as many unqualified.[1] The Medical Register was a voluntary listing compiled by Simmons for 1779, 1780 and 1783. For all three years the Long Buckby listing was Hubert and Anthony Floyer and Edward Swinfen.[2] I am greatly indebted to him for perusing these Registers for me.

Presumably Samuel Swinfen Harris had not yet come on the scene.

Qualification must have become more stringent with the examinations of 1815. The apothecaries had created a separate Company in 1616 but had been compelled to work under, and be supervised by, the physicians. As the physicians were relatively few in number – and only practised in London, larger cities and important places – the apothecaries were, for the most part, on their own and working as G.P.s. By the Apothecaries' Act, 1815, the Society of Apothecaries was allowed to supervise the training of, and examine, its own members. Training was by apprenticeship and the Licentiate of the Society of Apothecaries awarded. About 1815, also, the Royal College of Surgeons in London, established by Charter in 1800, created the grade of Membership for those other than hospital surgeons. So after 1815 many practitioners opted for the double qualification and, after 5 - 7 years apprenticeship, took their examinations in London and, if successful, qualified M.R.C.S., L.S.A. This made them Surgeon-Apothecaries, the qualification known as 'College and Hall'.

What was the nature of medical practice in the 18th Century? The short answer is that it was very competitive. Most of the work was visiting; distance appeared to be no object and, as journeys were undertaken mostly on horseback in all weathers, it was hard work. I have no doubt they gave a good service. Apothecaries, ipso facto, dispensed probably with ways and means of getting medicines out to patients, taking them out with them, delivering when riding nearby or dispensing from their panniers. The reason for the competition locally was that there was no agreed restrictive practice area.

References:

1. Transported to New South Wales: medical convicts 1788 - 1850, David Richards, *British Medical Journal, Volume 295,* 19th - 26th December 1987.
2. Personal communication from Dr. David Richards, Head, Department of Social Studies, School of Human Sciences, Trent Polytechnic, Nottingham.

SACRED to the memory of
EDWARD SWINFEN Surgeon,
By a constant and unremitting attention to
the discharge of his professional duties,
by his urbanity and benevolence,
He secur'd the confidence and esteem
of an extensive and respectable connection
To the poor he was a friend and benefactor
ever ready to alleviate their distress
by his advice and assistance
This monument also perpetuates the memory of
ANN SWINFEN (Mother of the above,
A native of Newbold in LEICESTERSHIRE)
Who favour'd with the enjoyment of her faculties
far beyond the usual period,
closed a well spent life in the firm hope of
a happy immortality
Also MARY HARRIS,
much beloved and respected wife of
and daughter and sister
of the above

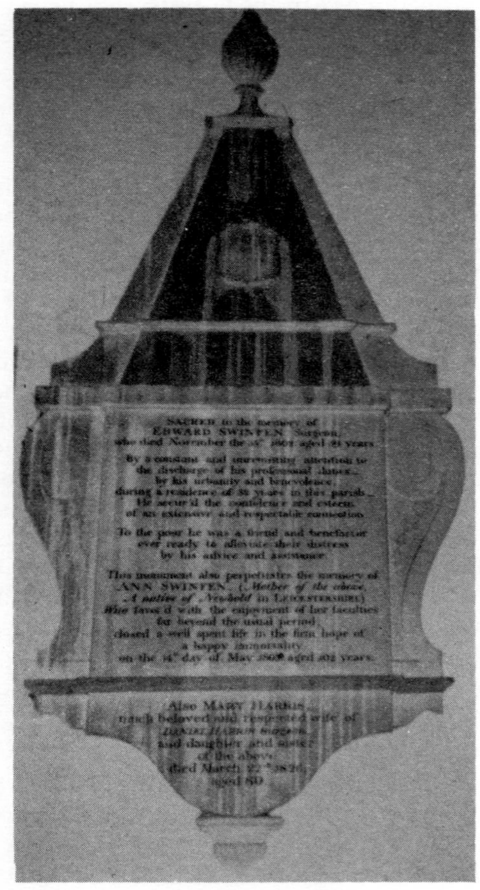

Monument to Dr. Swinfen in the church of St. Lawrence, Long Buckby.

I have recently been privileged to see a map prepared from known patients' addresses and giving, therefore, all the parishes visited by the Heygates' practice – father and son – West Haddon contemporaries of Floyer and Swinfen. They visited all the parishes visited by the two practices – not even allowing the Long Buckby apothecaries a monopoly in their own parish – and numerous additional ones. Their practice area was, therefore, considerably larger than the writer's modern practice covered by motor car. Likewise they would have been in competition with practitioners in Market Harborough, Guilsborough (if a practice) and south west of the Watling Street (the modern A5) which with the exception of the parishes of Kilsby and Ashby St. Ledgers, was not crossed by the West Haddon apothecaries. One wonders whether there was a tacit agreement between the Daventry apothecaries and the West Haddon practice to make the Watling Street a dividing line between spheres of interest. If this were the case the Long Buckby practices would probably have been limited to the East of the road also.

It was mostly private practice as it was a little too early in most country districts for Friendly Societies. The Appothecaries might, however, have begun to run their own 'clubs' towards the end of the 18th Century. There was a limited amount of paternalism as evidenced by Edward Sabin's (Towcester) day book. So aristocracy and gentry might have paid for medical attention to their chief servants – domestic and estate – and even to their huntsmen. The other source of income, which was lucrative, was appointment to attend the paupers of the parishes. As Poor Relief was on a Parish basis there was great scope for an energetic apothecary. Payment for this work was of two sorts. In parishes with very small populations the apothecary was mostly paid per item of service and for medicines given as was Edward Swinfen at Brington – although it was not an unduly small parish. The other mode of payment was by stipend. As we shall see in the 19th Century the Long Buckby doctors were paid an agreed (mostly on the Vestry's side!) annual salary. An account of Edward Swinfen's to the Overseers of the Poor of Brington 1784/85 is extant. He charged 2s-6d for riding to Brington, did not always visit but obviously always dispensed for a described condidion, often more than one medicament. For only 2 journeys, dressings to leg on one occasion, medicines, repeat prescriptions on 10 dates in 9 months his bill amounted to £2-4s-4d. Not bad remuneration though to be fair I think 8s-6d of that was an outstanding account, but he wasn't troubled very much by the two villages in the parish over that nine-month period.

Reference:

1. Heygate practice Map prepared by Mrs. J. M. Raybould for the West Haddon Local History Group. (West Haddon parish adjoins Long Buckby).

So the overall impression is that the apothecaries made a good living if they worked hard, and most did. Edward Swinfen was a good business man, efficient, methodical, a man of affairs – they were all men of affairs – and meticulous in his itemization of an account to a Brington family which had had a lot of illness in several members of the household. This was 1779/80, an account that had been allowed to run on for 10 months, all in his own handwriting. He obviously entered things in a day book or in patients'/families'[1] running accounts day by day. Incidentally he did not charge extra for a night journey to Brington; it was still 2s-6d.[2] Judged by Hubert Floyer's land investments I am sure he had the same attributes and business acumen as Edward Swinfen. A visit to 'The Chantry', Edward Jenner's home from 1785 to 1823, in Berkeley, Gloucestershire, gives one a good idea of the late 18th Century/early 19th Century apothecary's life of style and of a certain affluence.

What clinical work did they do? This can only be conjectured. There was no line on run-of-the-mill illness at Northamptonshire County Record Office. The prosperity of the village in the 18th Century depended on woolcombing and worsted-weaving, yet the Wellcome Institute for the History of Medicine disappointingly came up with nothing about these cottage industries. I was hoping for some references on woolsorter's disease and anthrax.

Victor Hatley says the work was unhealthy but does not elaborate. "In order to keep the wool flexible, the combs had to be heated by charcoal stoves which were known as 'comb pots'. The fumes given out by these stoves were noxious, and woolcombing was an unhealthy occupation".[3] Presumably, therefore, the woolcombing fraternity had more than its share of respiratory disease. Bronchitis, asthma and the ever-present Pulmonary Tuberculosis would have been common while chills, lobar pneumonia and pleurisy might well have been prevalent due to draughts from doors and windows opened to let out the fumes and heat. Hot, stripped, sweating men; well, perhaps not stripped in the 18th Century, but with only a shirt, sitting outside the comb shop in a cool breeze eating their dinner would have been prey to chills and bronchitis or worse. Similarly going home after work, hot and scantly clad in all weathers, without first pausing to put on a coat, would have predisposed to chest infection.

Neither the Borough of Daventrie (sic) in the late 18th Century (Thomas Swinfen, Gentleman, Coroner of our Lord the King) Coroner's Inquisitions nor admissions to the General Infirmary at Northampton shed any light on Long Buckby morbidity. If the death was not by accident, drowning, suicide but was sudden or otherwise unexplained there was an Inquisition on view of the body.

References:

1. Reference, Northamptonshire Record Office, in manuscript.
2. Reference, Northamptonshire Record Office, in manuscript. His writing is easy to read.
3. 'Blaze' at Buckby: A note on a Forgotten Northamptonshire Industry, Victor A. Hatley. Northamptonshire Past and Present, vol iv, No.2. 1967/8.

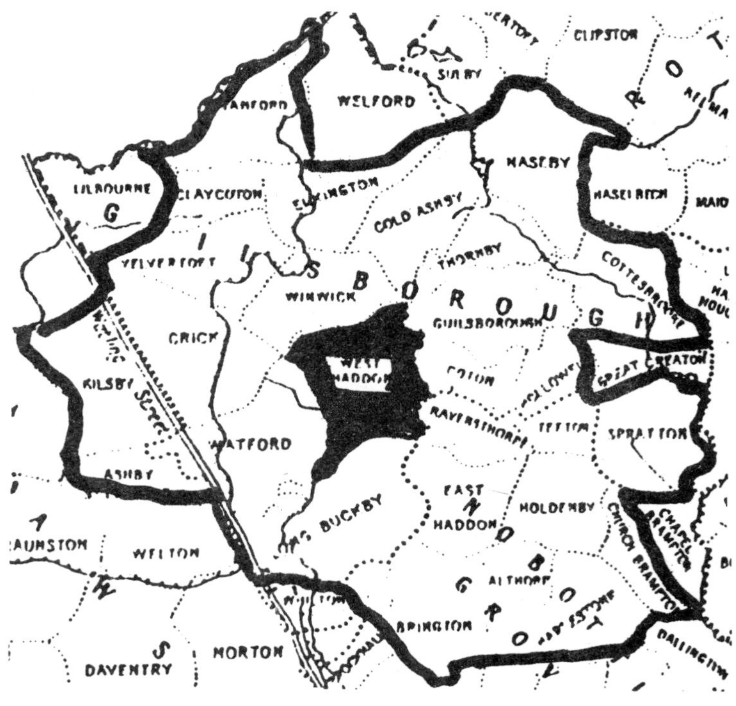

That part of Northamptonshire covered by the practice.

Thereafter, if there were no marks of violence appearing on the body, the person was deemed to have died by the visitation of God in a natural way and not otherwise. It was recorded on one occasion "...was in an extreem (sic) ill state of bodily health and so continued to languish, and languishing, did live until the eighteenth day of September..." which was not very specific.

Only six patients from Long Buckby were admitted to Northampton General Infirmary between 1743 and 1759. The diagnoses were Ulcering of the leg; Fever; Sorefoot; Sore leg and Obstructions. The principal causes of admission between 1743 and 1790 were ulcers, fevers, rheumatism, coughs, tumours and scurvy. Also mentioned were dropsy, eruptions and various accidental injuries. The diagnosis was given in virtually all in-patient cases from 1743 to 1780, then in half the cases between 1780 and 1790, thereafter progressively less.

What sort of men were they? Hubert Floyer married in 1753 but the date of his arrival is unknown. Whether he took over from Thomas West or another apothecary or set up on his own is not known. He was a shrewd man and it has been suggested to me that he might be regarded as an early land speculator. He started by owning property in Long Buckby, West Haddon and Denton. If one were not already a landed or moneyed person and one was looking to land as an investment, an easy and relatively cheap way of beginning to buy land was to purchase cottages to which belonged 'Cow Commons or Common of pasture (1 or 2 cows) in common fields'. And the cow commons could be sold away from the cottage and bought independently of the property. If this sort of transaction were done in several parishes in the years before Inclosure the investor could expect an award of land at the Inclosure of these parishes. As the value of land nearly doubled in value after inclosure the investor realised a handsome profit.[1] He bought property in Long Buckby in 1764; he also bought several other pieces of land in the next two years. Long Buckby's Inclosure was 1765. Floyer received two allotments: one of 3 acres 3 roods -perches and another of 4 acres 1 rood and 23 perches, the annual value of which was £10-16s-3d. He contributed £4-10s-6d towards the cost of the Inclosure Act, 1765.[2] The indentures for his West Haddon land or property purchases have not been found but he acquired land in the same way as at Long Buckby. West Haddon Inclosure was 1764 and he was awarded 35 acres 2 roods 122 perches in lieu of half a yard of land and Right of Common thereto belonging; worth £15-10s-6d. How much half a yard of land in this context is not known.

References:

1. Hubert Floyer, YZ 877 NRO, 18.6.1765 Indenture Release (i.e. Sale). Wm Darnell, Long Buckby, oatmeal maker, oldest son and heir of John Darnell, late of Long Buckby, to Hubert Floyer, Surgeon, Long Buckby for £18 of 3 Cow Commons or Common of Pasture for 3 cows in common fields.
2. Source:- Long Buckby Inclosure Award 1766.

Again at Denton (Inclosure 1770) "to the said Hubert Floyer Owner of one yard of Land and a half and three Cottages Commons and the right of Common thereto belonging and in lieu thereof The Two following Plots of Land or Ground, that is to say One Plot of Land lying and being in the said Fields called the Wood..." his award amounted to 3 acres 2 roods and 34 perches. He must have sold this before he died because it is not mentioned in his will.

One finds indentures to his name (YZ 865 NRO) 27.12 1765:
Indenture released (i.e. sale):

(1) John Robinson Long Buckby, Flaxdresser, to Hubert Floyer,
(2) for £112-10s-6d of moiety or half part of two half quarters in Long Buckby. (i.e. '18th of one yard of land).

There is mention of premises (which?) in a Bond in £215 (YZ 888 N.R.O., 21.2.1766). Hubert Floyer to enjoy premises released (sold) to him without let. The Bond was only forfeit if the conditions of the agreement were broken. He had a fair amount of land in the parish as will be realised by another indenture and by the fact that the family owned a small farm of 60 acres known to this day as Floyer's farm. Whether he bought 60 acres or whether later owners added to it is uncertain. Indenture Mortgage 1.11.1780 (YZ 915, N.R.O.) (1) Hubert Floyer to (2) Wm Biggs, the Younger, Welford carrier for £400 of new (clearly built it) dwelling house, garden etc., and 3 new inclosures called Newland, Codwell and Narborough (14 acres) – two allotted at Inclosure and one bought of John Lee. A mortgage of this size indicates a large house and a good land holding.

Unfortunately he was to enjoy his new house for less than a year. He died the next year having made a will on 10th April which was proved on 14th September 1781. In it the life interest in the Long Buckby estate was left to the widow, and Anthony, the eldest son and heir at law, received the reversion of the whole messuage in Long Buckby. The Denton estate was divided between Anthony's younger brother William, also an apothecary, and his three sisters.

Anthony Floyer returned to the village after apprenticeship in 1775 or '76 in time to be included in the 1777 Militia List. He would have joined his father in practice during his father's last years. He had everything going for him – a ready-made practice with the goodwill built up over the years by his father, a fine house, an assured position and the whole of his father's estate in Long Buckby coming to him on his mother's death – but it was not to be.

Perhaps the following indenture is an omen of what was to come. Anthony Floyer YZ 885 N.R.O. 1777. An agreement between Anthony Floyer, surgeon and apothecary, and his mother respecting the use of chemicals, board and lodging etc. The father had not died then; the chemicals were his and were pharmaceuticals used in the practice. Did Mary Floyer well know her husband as soft-hearted regarding Anthony? Was Anthony already a bit of a harum-scarum and could not be trusted to keep a gentleman's agreement, so it was put down in writing? Or was she a grasping, hard-nosed woman?

The reasons for his failure in life were probably several. These can only be hazarded as conjectures and certainly cannot all be substantiated as fact. First his father's will – he did not enter into his inheritance until his mother's death and that was 20 years later – secondly personal and family difficulties which may be hinted at in his colleague's very detailed will. Fair enough his mother should have been provided for but was he expected to pay the housekeeping expenses and keep his mother and sisters despite his mother having an income from the land? She might have asserted her position as head of the family and owner of the house until her death, but neither she nor the estate paid off the £400 mortgage. So Anthony not only inherited the estate after his mother's death he also inherited his father's £400 mortgage to help pay for his new house in 1780 and, as this was not repaid, his father's Bond in £800, 1780 YZ 921 N.R.O. 1.11.1780. Bond in £800. Hubert Floyer to Wm Biggs, the Younger, Welford, Carrier, to pay £400 secured by indenture. This meant that he would forfeit the bond of £800 if he did not repay the £400 morgage to Wm Biggs. So perhaps his financial position for the 20 years after his father's death was not as rosy as he and everyone else supposed. No doubt he would have been allowed credit on his expectations which became increasingly far distant. Having said all this, he did have a well established practice and should have had an adequate income. So perhaps a weakness of character exhibited itself. Perhaps he enjoyed country pursuits and preferred hunting to practising. It is known that a pack of harriers was kept in Long Buckby around this time by Geo Freeman Esq., son of the Rev. Dr. Freeman, The vicar. Hunting can be expensive. He was still a bachelor and the company he mixed with may have had more money than him. There would have been many who wished to be friendly with the sporting doctor. He may well have been extravagant; unfortunately his means did not allow him to live in the style to which he intended to become accustomed. He certainly showed no foresight. He must have known he would have to repay the £400 mortgage yet no attempt was made to do this from income before his mother died; indeed it was not paid off until 1810.

He married Sarah Wood, spinster, of the parish of Long Buckby by licence on 23-iv-1807. She could only make her mark. He was 50-52 years of age.

After his mother's death and coming into the estate he must have thought matters would improve but things had probably gone too far. He mortgaged land (?), called a messuage etc. in Long Buckby for £250 in 1807. Then in 1810 there was Assignment and Ratification of Anthony Floyer's Mortgage of an estate in Long Buckby. His wife was involved. She again could only make her mark. All others party to the deed could sign their names. What sort of woman was she? As Mrs. Floyer was party to the deed it suggests she had a legal interest in the property. Was it part (or all) of her marriage settlement?

The state his affairs were in resulted in the two following indentures:

Anthony Floyer YZ 879 N.R.O. 17.11.1810.

Indenture Released (i.e. sale)

(1) Anthony Floyer, Long Buckby, Surgeon and Apothecary, eldest son and heir of Hubert Floyer, Wm Cooper, Long Buckby, Yeoman.

(2) Joshua Cure, Long Buckby, Yeoman.

(3) Wm. Sergeant Denny, Long Buckby, Gent (a solicitor) and John Robinson of Broadway Lane, Long Buckby, Grazier.

To pay off mortgage to Wm. Biggs, Welford, Yeoman, of £400 secured by mortgage from Hubert Floyer to Wm. Biggs his father of 1st November 1780. To pay off Samuel Walker of West Haddon Lodge, Gent, of £250 (that was only a 3 years old Indenture Mortgage).

To raise a further £150 from (2)

Now (1) with consent of (2) to (3) as Trustees of messuage and yard in Long Buckby, 3 closes called Newland Codwell, and Narborough (14 acres), 2 allotted to Hubert Floyer at inclosure and one purchased of John Lee.

To sell same and pay off £800 if the same is not repaid...

Anthony Floyer YZ 882 N.R.O. 17.11.1810.
Mortgage Bond in £1400
Anthony Floyer to Joshua Cure, Long Buckby, Gent to repay £800.

The final blow fell in 1816 (YZ 920 N.R.O. 1816). There is a sad document in Anthony's handwriting: "I have this Noon March 5th 1816 sold to my Brother Wm Floyer all my Land, Home and Freehold and other appurtenances thereunto belonging; upon condition that my Brother Wm Floyer discharge the Mortgage and all Interest due upon the said Estate; and hereafter pay to me during my natural life an Annuity of £30 per annum and the liberty at my pleasure to live in the said Home free of rent during my future life – in testimony of which contract and bargain – we have hereunto each of us affixed our names.

Signed: *A. Floyer*
Wm. Floyer

Anthony had certainly come down in the world. In 1815 he could not even afford a horse. He may have been lent one but he did not own one as he was not taxed for a horse. He and Wm. Dix were the only two apothecaries listed in the tax returns for the year 5th April 1814 to the 5th April 1815. Anthony's house had 11 windows, more than most. There was one house each of 13 and 14 windows, 3 of 11 windows, 5 of 10 while most had 6 windows including Dix's. Others less.

Anthony's practice could not have been much without a horse. It must have been confined to the village – or as far as he cared to walk – and to those patients who were prepared to come to him.

Who followed him is uncertain.

Edward Swinfen was a character. Described if not quite in hyperbole, at least in glowing terms on his church tablet, he died at the comparatively early age of 59 years in 1802. Born therefore in 1743, he came to the village in 1770 and practised here for 32 years. One cannot help wondering whether some of the urbanity and benevolence mentioned owed something to smugness and self satisfaction. It rather seems he did not have a great deal of conscientious competition from the other practice. In comparison it would be easy. "...To the poor he was a friend and benefactor ever ready to alleviate their distress by his advice and assistance". "By a constant and unremitting attention to the discharge of his professional duties...". This is not to detract from his professional achievements. As we have seen he was no slouch on the business side, being methodical and carefully accurate, so I am sure, had he not been conscientious, he would not have been doctor to the Poor at Brington and probably in two or three other parishes as well.

This monument records his mother's notable achievement of reaching 102 years and who died the year after him. It also shows that this was a medical family, his sister having married Daniel Harris, a surgeon.

He did well in 32 years of practice.

He owned his house and with it approaching half the centre of the village, then called the Mount and now lying between King Street and Church Street. The Mounts are now thought of as a slight rise with a modern bungalow on the site near Sibley House. His house stood on the site of Castle House (No. 12 King Street). In view of the disastrous fire in Surgeon Harris's time I don't suppose the present house represents much, if anything, of the original building.

He owned land mentioned in his Will as Homers Leys (presumably Hammers Leys), land in Ravensthorpe and was involved with Thomas Swinfen, of Daventry, Plumber and Glazier, in buying and selling property in Daventry and Drayton. So with one or two exceptions they were all at it. Thomas Swinfen was brother of Edward and in another context, Coroner of Daventry Borough, Gent.

Swinfen never married. He had a large family of nephews and nieces as one discovers by reading his very detailed "D.I.Y." Will running to 9 larger-than-A4 sheets in his own handwriting. It is an impressive document drawn up about 3 months before he died; neat, legible and in a firm hand which makes such a lengthy manuscript all the more remarkable. It must have saved quite a lot in legal fees. What Mr. Wm. S. Denny, lawyer, thought when he was asked to sign this last Will and Testament as one of the three witnesses is anybody's guess. He was obviously very family minded. He looked after his mother – was at pains to leave her well provided for after his death and for her lifetime – cared for his sister and a niece and seemed to want to share his worldly success in terms of possesions, land, property and money, after realization of assets, round the family. But he was shrewd and hard-headed. The length and scrupulosity of his Will were, I think, partly occasioned by his large family, the special circumstances of two of them, and partly deriving from long, observant Floyer – watching. The main provision was an income of £30 of lawful Money of the United Kingdom of Great Britain and Ireland p.a., out of his estate for his mother during the term of her natural life. After her death his estate was to be made chargeable with the payment of one other annuity, or Clear Yearly Rent Charge, of £10.

This was to be paid unto his niece Ann Maria Stanton, wife of Thomas Stanton, during the term of her natural life, and for her sole only and Proper Use and Benefit in some Inn or Public House in Long Buckby by the aforesaid, in equal quarterly payments. This seems to mean she was to enjoy the annuity and spend it as she liked; certainly it was intended for her use only. "...and wherewith the said Thomas Stanton shall have no...,(indecipherable) meddling or concern nor shall the same be subject to the Debts or Controle (sic) of the said Thomas Stanton in any way whatsoever." Swinfen knew his man.

The main beneficiary was his nephew Samuel Swinfen Harris, Surgeon. For his lifetime he owned the Messuage in Long Buckby, Hammer's Leys; he received Swinfen's horses, his hay, all his Stock-in-Trade, Tinctures, Drugs, Instruments and whatever appertained to his profession of a Surgeon, Appothecary (sic) and midwife and also all my household goods – he permitting (sic) his mother (Swinfen's sister Mary Harris) to take such part thereof, not exceeding in value £20, as she shall think proper. He shared the linen with his mother. But he received all Swinfen's clothes, all the china, a silver tankard and the best of the plate (silver). There were several bequests of individual items of silver.

Samuel Swinfen Harris was to give Swinfen's mother uninterupted residence in his house during her life. He was also directed to give his mother, Mary Harris, residence therein during her life unless "my said sister and my nephew Samuel Swinfen Harris shall choose to live apart then, in such case, I do hereby Will and direct that my said nephew, Samuel Swinfen Harris, shall fit up in a neat and comfortable manner the room adjoining my best parlor (sic) and the room over the same as a residence for my said sister, Mary Harris his mother, during her life and my mind and Will is that in that case my said Nephew shall pay all Taxes and Levys for the same and also keep the same in repare (sic) during my said sister Mary Harris's life."

It would be tedious to detail all the bequests after property and land had been sold. He left property to his Sister Mary. "If however her husband, Daniel Harris, were to show up and claim an interest in the said premises then the said Devise was to be made void and the property was to be given and devised to his Trustees. She was then to get the Rents, Issues and Profits after deducting for repairs during the term of her Natural Life to and for her own Use and Benefit free from the Debts and Controls of the said Daniel Harris and wherewith he shall have no meddling or controle."

Yes, I think his will depicts him as a character but as an essentially nice, warm-hearted family man. Great fun at home I shouldn't wonder – very avuncular. Piquancy is added at the end of the Will when our paragon directs his Trustees to purchase 12 rings, the same to be given to my said Brother etc"..."the last to be given unto my esteemed friend Mrs. Henrietta Maria Iliff."

Little is known of Samuel Swinfen Harris other than that he was Edward Swinfen's heir, lived in his house and practised from that address. It seems likely that his disastrous fire in 1810 compelled either his immediate or early retirement. Certainly he was not practising in 1814 when the Tax Returns for 5th April 1814 to 5th April 1815 listed Anthony Floyer and Wm. Dix as the only two apothecaries in the village. This Document makes it almost proof positive that Dix followed Harris. Harris died in 1818.

Harris's fire was a different one from the calamitous fire of 1814 which broke out in Bluckley's Plough manufactory and partly consumed 7 houses and outhouses (N.M. 18th June 1814) Reference (1). 2nd List Individuals in many surrounding parishes contributed to the distress fund.

But the latter half of the 18th Century with Hubert Floyer coming to the end of his career, Anthony young and full of promise, Edward Swinfen in his prime and the West Haddon practice coming into the parish, some thought there was still room for another practitioner. Wm. March, the elder, Weaver, in a will made on 28th February 1783, proved in Northampton 23rd April 1792..."I give and bequeath unto my son, Thomas, all my 4 looms with the Implements thereto belonging, my Warping Mill with the Tackle, my Grinding Wheel with all things appertaining thereto, my Shaving Bleeding and Tooth – Drawing Instruments, also my Wearing Apparel...". So, in addition to this surely being the earliest reference to dentistry in Long Buckby, we had a quack plying his (part-time?) trade as a Barber-Surgeon. Weaving would not have been so lucrative by this date.

2. 19th Century Doctors

Were it not for the preservation of the Long Buckby Vestry Minutes for the years 1826 to 1844 the beginning of this part of my account would be even sketchier than it is. However, the succession from the 18th to the 19th Century Practitioners is largely conjectural as is the succession from one to another, especially in one of the practices, in the second and third decades of the 19th Century. It all gets easier when various Directories are available for scrutiny from 1830. Maddeningly Pigot's London and Provincial New Commercial Directory, 1839, only lists the surgeons of one practice. The gap of 10 years before it reappears on the reference shelves misses a doctor known from another source and prevents proof of the assumption that he was in opposition to the aforementioned practitioners.

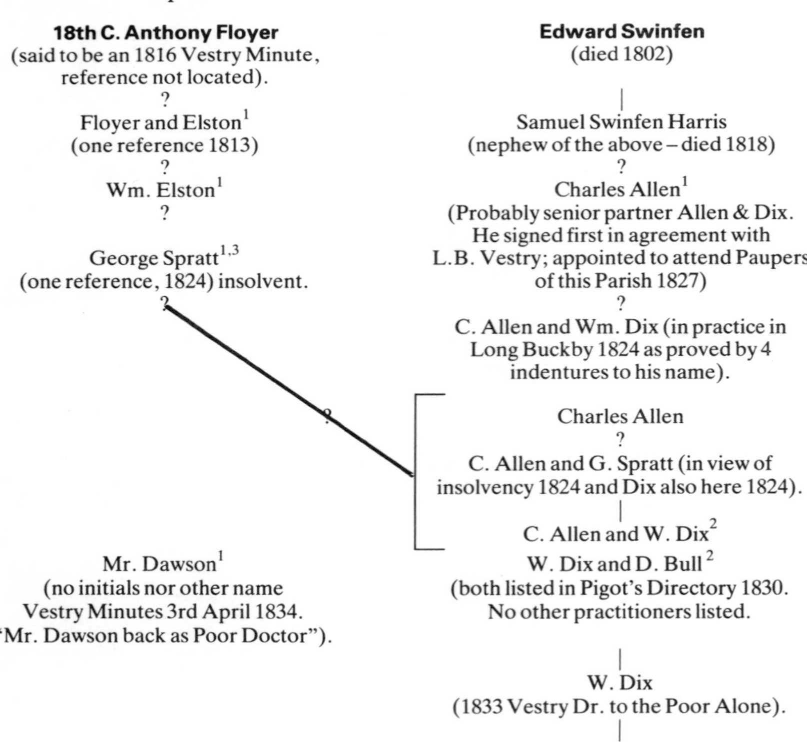

Dawson
?
Henry Scrase (first listed in Pigot's Directory, 1840, alone in 1841 & 1847 Directories.

H. Scrase and Wm. Watson first listed (Whellan's 1849).

W. Watson (umarried), listed as one of two Principals 1851 census Study.[5] So Scrase has retired.

Private residents Wm. Watson Surgeon listed below under Commercial. 1854 Kelly's Directory. Wm. Watson, Surgeon (retired 1858).

Arthur Cox (1858)

Private Cox, Arthur Esq., Commercial, Cox, Arthur Surgeon — P.O. Directory 1864[6]

Wm. Dicks (sic)[4] listed alone in 1840, 1841, 1847 and 1849. His qualification becomes M.D. 1849 Whellan's & Kelly's Directories.

W. Dix (assisted by his son Frederick)[5] and his other son William (? also called Andrew)

Kelly's Directory 1854. Private Residents Wm. Dix M.D. listed below under Commercial Wm. Dix & Sons Surgeons.

Private Dix, Wm. M.D. Commercial Dix, Wm. & Son Surgeons

(Wm. Dix died on 29th October 1865 aged 77 years).

2 single handed Practices.

(Private) Cox Arthur (Commercial) — Kelly's Directory 1877 — (Private) Commercial) Frederick Wm. Dix.

Arthur Cox — Kelly's Direc. 1885
Private Residents Cox, Arthur High Street.
Commerical Cox, Arthur Surgeon Holly House, High Street, Long Buckby.
Kelly 1890 – Surgeon, Medical Officer and Public Vaccinator No. 4 District, Daventry Union.

Cox & Son

Not certain when Arthur Cox retired. Died 1st February 1909.

Frederick Wm. Dix
Private Resident,
Churchouse, Wm. John Franklin. High Sreet, Long Buckby.
Dix, Frederick Wm., High Street, Long Buckby.
Commercial, Churchouse Wm. J. Franklin L.R.C.P. Edin. Surgeon (firm of Dix & Churchouse).
Dix, Frederick Wm., (firm of Dix & Churchouse), Surgeon & Medical Officer, Public vaccinator, 5th District Brixworth Union.

Churchouse came to Long Buckby in 1883

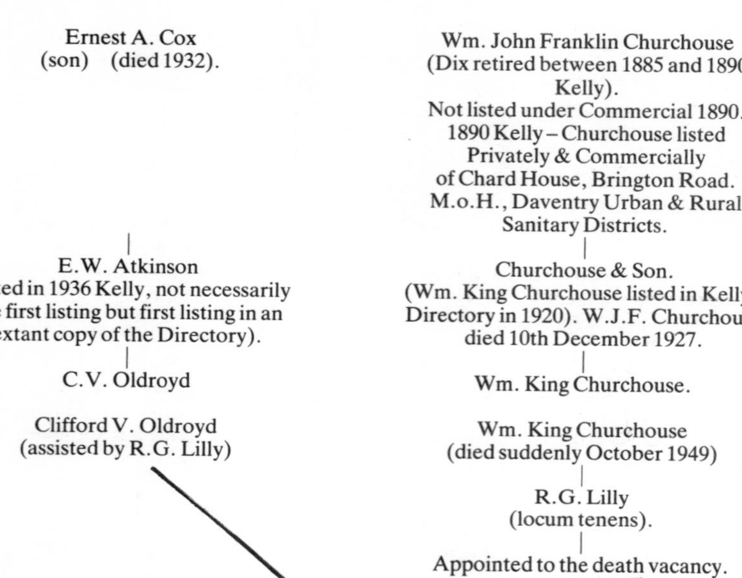

End of October 1949

Clifford Oldroyd and Graham Lilly
(assisted at first by E.A.C. (Nan) Thomson).

Graham Lilly and Norman How.

Norman How and Graham Craddock.

References:

1. = 1 reference practitioners.
2. = 3 reference practitioners,
3. Long Buckby Baptisms Register 1813-1874.

Baptised	*Born*	*Name*	*Parents*	*Surname*	*Abode*	*Trade/Prof.*
June 21st 1824	18.1.1820	Julia	George	Spratt	L. Buck	Surgeon
June 21st 1824	24.4.1824	Louisa	Maria	Spratt	"	Surgeon

Found after this section had been written.

4. Wm. Dix M.D., Erlangen 1840. In practice before 1815 (L.S.A.) Act. Member of the Council of the Provincial Medical and Surgical Association. Medical Directory 1847 (first) Edition.
5. The Population of a Northamptonshire Village 1851. A Census Study of Long Buckby (Vaughan Paper No. 16, University of Leicester Dept. of Adult Education).
6. P.O. Directory, Northants., Hunts., Beds., Berks., Bucks. and Oxon.

What can be said of these men? Well; very little of the four one – reference men and one three – reference man. William Elston's existence is only known by a reference in Northamptonshire Record Office that, in 1813, he signed a certificate exempting a man service with the Militia on health grounds...[1] News of George Spratt's bankruptcy appeared in the Northampton Mercury in 1824. Which 'side' these two fit in is conjectural. Charles Allen is mentioned in the Long Buckby Vestry Minutes 1827. "We the undersigned agree to undertake the medical and surgical attendance of the paupers of this parish for the sum of £36 p.a., exclusive of all journeys out of the parish·"

Signed CHARLES ALLEN.   Wm DIX. Surgeons[2]

The fact that Allen signed first makes it almost certain he was senior partner. 'Mr.' Dawson is interesting in that the wording of the Vestry Minute makes it almost certain that he was in opposition to Dix and Bull, or Dix alone, and that there was competition for the appointment of medical attendants of the paupers. "Mr. Dawson back as Doctor at £35 p.a."[3] D. Bull was junior partner to Dix and they were joint parish doctors in 1830 at a fee of £30 p.a.[4]

Although I think the doctors were keen to be the Parish Doctor, but not at any price. In 1832 Bull and his senior partner declined an offer of the medical duties of the parish at £35 p.a.[5] This must have provoked a crisis because, the post having been given to an outside doctor, it is obvious that there was solidarity between the two Long Buckby practices regarding what they considered suitable remuneration for the appointment. On the 10th April 1832 Mr. Edward Swan of Weedon was appointed for the ensuing year, his duties to include Midwifery, Small Pox (sic) and Accidents.[6] Whether Small Pox meant attendance on cases of smallpox or vaccination is not certain; very possibly both. It could not have been a very satisfactory arrangement. Even though Weedon would have been 4½ to 5 miles away by bridle path, compared with 6 miles by modern road, it was a long way for the doctor to come. And it must have been very hard work for him, 'hacking' across to Buckby in all weathers, most days of the week and at all times of day and night (N.B. midwifery).

References:

1. The L.S.A. listings show the residence, (?) at date of qualification – William Alfred Elston, Brigbrooke (sic) 1833 so he was either practising unqualified or was apprenticed to a Buckby doctor when he exempted a man Militia Service – more likely the latter. The 1848 Medical Directory lists A.W. Elston and W.H. Walker (P.L.M.O. Northampton Union) at Bugbrooke.
2. Long Buckby Vestry Minutes, 6 April 1827.
3. Ibid. 3 April 1834.
4. Ibid. 8 April 1830.
5. Ibid. 1 April 1832.
6. Ibid. 10 April 1832.

Small wonder that Dix got the job again next year. "Mr. Dix (alone) got the medical attendance contract back at £35 p.a.[1] They did not get quite what they wanted (£36 p.a., in 1827) but £35 was better than the £30 fee of 1830 so the cut was nearly restored. Mr. Dawson's appointment at £35 p.a., next year was presumably the last time in view of the Poor Law Amendment Act 1834. So it seems that both the doctors and the Vestry settled for £35 for the last few years of the Parish Doctor System.

While it may seem that the doctors had to fight for their fees and there may be sympathy that their zeal and professional skill were not recompensed by adequate remuneration, it has to be pointed out that their highest recorded fee of £35 p.a. coincided with the highest amount then spent on the poor (£2,073). The annual amount spent on the poor from then until 1834 always topped £2,000 and reached an unprecedented height of £2,798 in 1832, the year the doctors were battling hard for £36 p.a., and the Vestry was trying its best to hold down expenditure on the poor. Somehow it did because it 1833 only £2,282 was spent. All this has to be seen against a backgound of extreme poverty, rising population (1,600 in 1801 to 2,145 in 1841 and higher), the collapse of the flourishing woolcombing and worsted-weaving industry in the 1790s and the yet to be fully established shoe trade.

The first major figure of the 19th Century was William Dix. Born in 1788, after partnership first with Charles Allen and then with Dr. Bull, he was single-handed from about 1833 (sole Parish doctor) until 1850 or so (evidence of Directories 1840-1849 when his name was spelt Dicks). He can be traced locally at the age of 36 by four indentures to his name at the County Records office. This was 1824.[2] The 1851 Census lists him[3] as assisted by his sons Frederick and William, who was probably also called Andrew and who was only, I think, apprenticed to him. However, in 1854 he was definitely in partnership with his son Frederick William and Kelly's Directory of that year records for the first time the higher degree of M.D.[4], a first for Long Buckby.

References:

1. Long Buckby Vestry Minutes, 4th April 1833.
2. The Collector's Duplicate of Taxes levied on the Several Inhabitants of L. Buckby for the year 5.4.1814 to 5.4.1815 lists Wm. Dix taxed on his own house of 6 windows, as employing a groom and owning a horse for private use. (Mrs. George Thompson's property).
3. The population of a Northamptonshire Village, 1851. A Census Study of L. Buckby (Vaughan Paper No. 16, University of Leicester, Dept. of Adult Education).
4. Medical Directory 1847 Edition (first) M.D. Erlangen 1840. In practice prior to Act of 1815 (Apothecaries Act – L.S.A.). Member of Council of the Provincial Medical and Surgical Association (forerunner of the B.M.A.). Contributor to Medical and Physical Journal of a paper on "penetrating wounds of the abdomen,, and to the Medical Gazette on "intestinal worms and bilary calculi" (1825).

That he never used this in Consultant Practice is shown by all the Kelly's and P.O. Directories until his death which listed, and still do until the latest one I have seen in 1920, the doctors and others under Private Residents – Wm. Dix M.D., and again under Commercial – Wm. Dix and Son, Surgeons. He died on 29th october 1865 aged 77 years, nominally in harness in Long Buckby, being listed in the P.O. Directory the year before he dies as a Private Resident as well as Commercially as Dix and Son, Surgeons. He was probably Surgeon, Medical Officer and Public Vaccinator of the 5th District of the Brixworth Union. His son was in 1885. This was a long time after 1834 and the creation of the Unions for it to be a first appointment.

Early in Dix's time, 1829, there is a Vestry Minute "Agreed to increase the annual subscription to the General Infirmary in Northampton (now known as Northampton General Hospital) from £5-5-0 to £7-7-0.[1]. Scrutiny of the early clinical records of the hospital does suggest that more patients from Long Buckby were dealt with after the parish subscription was raised. This would not be accounted for by midwifery. You were delivered successfully – or unsuccessfully – at home. So far as I know there was no specific maternity department at this early stage. There would still have been no point in admitting any patient with major or internal surgical disease. Lord Lister was not to be present at the first operation performed in England under ether anaesthesia until 1846. Chloroform was not to be used by Sir James Young Simpson in Edinburgh for obstetric purposes until 1847. Besides all this Lord Lister's publication of his antiseptic results for the three previous years was not to come out until 1867. When Dix was young amputation of a limb could be a fatal operation. Yet he would have tried to prevent death from sepsis in cases of severe compound fracture of a limb by admitting such cases to hospital. The journey on frightful roads with rough and ready horsedrawn transport would have been an ordeal indeed. At the cost of appalling suffering and pain, shock, possible haemorrhage and probably worsening of the condition there was no guarantee of forestalling infection. Despite distance, bad roads and primitive transport the Northampton Infirmary did not have long to wait for its first road accident casualty. Within a month of opening for the reception of patients on 29th March 1744 the *Northampton Mercury* of 23rd April 1744 reported that a boy fell under the wheels of a waggon he was driving at Stoke Goldington in Buckinghamshire, on the Newport Pagnell - Northampton turnpike, which crushed his foot in a terrible manner. Victor Hatley stated in a *memo* to the *Northamptonshire Past and Present* that perusal of the early hospital records show that he was discharged as "cured" on 7th July 1744 after in-patient treatment lasting for well over two months.

Waddy on page 34 of his book[2] states that in 1835 the number of beds had to be increased to 112 because of the number of serious accidents brought in from the work of construction of the London and Birmingham Railway particularly at Blisworth and Kilsby. These consisted of severe simple and compound fractures, dislocations and lacerated wounds.

Small wonder there were so many casualties when we read Terry Coleman's graphic account of the railway navvies – their conditions of work, their roughness, their drunkenness, the danger, their riots and their recklessness.[3]

References:

1. Long Buckby Vestry Minutes, 1st March 1829.
2. Waddy, F.F., A History of Northampton General Hospital, 1743 to 1948, *The Guildhall Press (Northampton) Limited,* 1974.
3. Coleman, Terry, The Railway Navvies, *Hutchinson & Co. (Publishers) Limited,* 1965.

There are two sets of figures, and causes of death in Northamptonshire Records:

Yearly Bill of Mortality Within the Parish of All Saints from 21st December 1850 to 21st December 1851.

Abscess	1	Childbed	1	Fever	3	Measles	2
Aged	13	Consumption	15	Hoop. Cough	1	Sc. Fever	2
Apoplexy	2	Convulsion	1	Inflammat.	12	Teeth	1
Asthma	1	Dis. in Heart	2	Insane	1	Water in Chest	2
Cancer	1	Dropsy	2	Jaundice	1	Destroyed himself by cutting his throat	1

Whereof have died.

Under 2 yrs.	17	Btwn. 10 & 20	1	Btwn. 40 & 50	2	Btwn. 70 & 80	7
Btwn. 2 & 5	3	Btwn 20 & 30	2	Btwn. 50 & 60	10	Btwn. 80 & 90	4
Btwn. 5 & 10	4	Btwn. 30 & 40	6	Btwn. 60 & 70	8	Btwn. 90 & 100	1

Total 65. The 17 deaths under 2 years represent 26% of the total.

The same Parish Yearly Bill of Mortality, 21st December 1851 to 21st December 1852.

Aged	12	Dis. in Heart	1	Palsy	1	Teeth	1
Asthma	2	Dropsy	1	Rupture	1	Typh. Fever	1
Consumption	9	Inflammation	8	Scalded	1	Ulcers	1
Convulsions	5	Measles	1	Suddenly	1	Water in Chest	1

Whereof have died.

Under 2 yrs.	14	Btwn. 10 & 20	2	Btwn. 40 & 50	2	Btwn. 70 & 80	8
Btwn. 2 & 5	3	Btwn. 20 & 30	3	Btwn. 50 & 60	2	Btwn. 80 & 90	1
Btwn. 5 & 10	1	Btwn. 30 & 40	4	Btwn. 60 & 70	7	Btwn. 90 & 100	0

Total 47. The 14 deaths under 2 years represents just less than 30% of the total.

From 1881 to 1900 there was no substantial improvement in the infant mortality in England and Wales, but from 1900 to 1927 the infant death rate (deaths of infants under 1 year of age) fell from 154 to 70 per 1,000 registered live - births per year.

While these Bills of Mortality are for a busy, town centre Parish in a large market and county town and, therefore, cannot be strictly comparable to the Parish of St. Lawrence, yet Dix would have treated much the same illness. Consumption (Pulmonary T.B.) was always with us; the infantile mortality was high everywhere; infectious disease now regarded as relatively mild could be fatal. Emergencies, heart disease and pleurisy could occur in town and country. But I cannot see Dix sending much of this sickness into hospital. So much for the medical side of things. Without surviving records of day to day work it is very difficult to get an accurate idea of the clinical content of general practice; and no such records exist. There is a wonderful reference in County Records – Dr. Edward Sabin (1751-1818) of Towcester's Day Book for the whole year, 1797-8. This, however, is not Long Buckby and it is 30 to 40 years before the time we are considering and so is not strictly comparable.

What of the man? I think it can be stated straightaway that he was a man of standing and probity; very probably comfortably off when he came to Long Buckby. Not long after his arrival having, presumably, bought a partnership, and a house, there are indentures assigning mortgages to Dix. He was, therefore, investing money by acting as mortgagee. He appears repeatedly in property deeds either as a mortgagee or as a trustee. There are no examples of his buying or selling property, as did the 18th Century apothecaries, for himself. This suggests either that any such deeds have not survived – unlikely in view of so many trustee etc., deeds surviving – or that he arrived in Long Buckby already well provided for. Having said that I did not find an indenture for the purchase of his own house. What is interesting is how he became widely known as a man prepared to act as a trustee or mortgagee. Parties in Elkington, Winwick, East Haddon; a party owning property in Daventry, Yelvertoft and Northampton; a co-trustee lived in Irthlingborough Parish, and he was involved at Flore and with people in Badby, Welford and distant parishes. This trustee work presumably attracted fees. An indenture of 1826 in which Dix was a party, but whose exact legal status is not clear, is interesting in that it has a consideration of no less than £1,187.10 shillings which, in 1826, must have been a very large sum of money, the price of a London house then.

Fredrick William Dix was born on the 14th December 1826 and died in December 1901 aged 74 years, a few days short of his 75th year and was buried on his birthday. He was living in retirement at the family home, and former practice house, in High Street, Long Buckby, being listed as a Private Resident at that address in the 1890 Kelly's Directory. Nothing is known of his schooling. He trained at University College, London, qualifying Member of the Royal College of Surgeons (M.R.C.S.) 1848, Licentiate of the Society of Apothecaries (L.S.A.) 1849. First mentioned in the 1851 Census as assistant to his father, when he would have been 25, he became his partner and later worked in single-handed practice from his father's death until 1883 – W.J.F. Churchouse's arrival. It would seem he was quietly content to follow in his father's professional footsteps though not in his trustee and business affairs. There are no legal references to his name at County Records. Content also to live in the same house for most of his life – certainly he died there – to work there and only to leave it, of necessity, for schooling and his medical education. That he went to boarding school is conjectural but almost certain. Whether the Old Daventry Grammar School was practical as a Day School I do not know.

He lived in the era of clinical horror and drama. Nothing more need be said about this because it is fully covered in the next section.

He and his family, or at least one of them, were I think men of their time. From scanty references it seems they took part in Victorian Associations for Social Improvement in Long Buckby. R.Dix, a younger brother, was on the Committee elected at the last A.G.M., of the Long Buckby Useful Knowledge Society.[1] Dix himself did a recitation at the 1st Annual Festival of the Long Buckby Mutual Improvement Society.[2] Whether he was truly interested in the Society's Lecture Programme or was merely inveigled into performing at the Annual Social Evening it is impossible to say. By taking part, though, he must have been tuned to the spirit of the times. Staunch Liberal and a Churchman, he practised for 40 years.

Of course, not the least of his achievements was to engage W.J.F. Churchouse as his assistant, later to become partner, in 1883.

Franklin Churchouse was born at Chard, Somerset, and educated at Chard Grammar School; he trained at Charing Cross Hospital and qualified Licentiate of the Society of Apothecaries, (L.S.A.) in 1879. Qualifying Licentiate of the Royal College of Physicians (L.R.C.P., Edinburgh) and Licentiate of the Royal Faculty of Physicians and Surgeons (L.R.F.P.S., Glasgow) in 1883. That he, a west countryman trained in London, should wish to add two Scottish Licentiates to his name must show in what high esteem the Scottish medical schools and licensing boards were then held. He was Demonstrator in Chemistry at Charing Cross Hospital and School.

"Dr. Churchouse was one of the most popular doctors in the county. For many years he was the regular medical attentant to the Spencer

Family and the "Red Earl" was so particularly attached to him that he often pressed him to stay at Althorp at nights. The deceased gentleman was greatly beloved for his kindness and genial courtesy and will be sadly missed in and around his home".[3]..."He was an officer in the old 'A' (Althorp) Coy of Volunteers under Capt. The Hon. C.R. Spencer as the late Earl then was. He was very keen on hunting before the war and whenever his professional duties allowed he enjoyed a gallop with the Pytchley."[3]

References:-

1. *Northampton Mercury,* 17th June 1854, by courtesy of Mr.R. Greenall, W.E.A., Long Buckby, 1988.
2. *Northampton Mercury,* 15th May 1872, by courtesy of Mr. R. Greenall W.E.A., Long Buckby, 1988.
3. Obituary, Dr. W.J.F. Churchouse, *The Northampton Independent,* 10th December 1927.

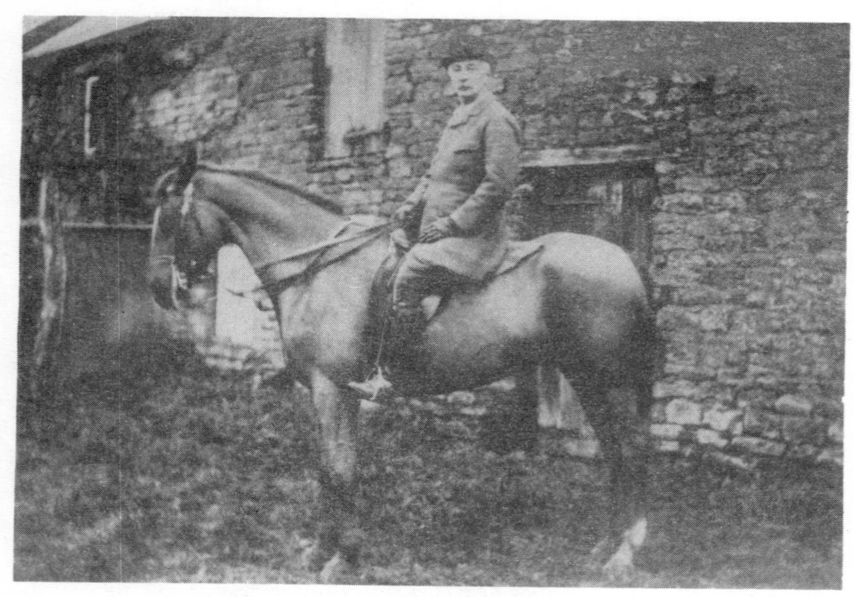

Dr. Franklin Churchouse

During the First World War he was in charge of the County Golf Links Hospital at Brampton; also of Lady Horne's hospital at East Haddon Institute and at Mrs. Guthrie's Hospital at East Haddon Hall. The combination of his former local authority experience, his war work and being the 'county' doctor meant that he had influence and could say a word in the right place. For 16 years since Churchouse's original initiative in trying to get a District Nurse, contributions to the funds of Long Buckby Nursing Association had been painstakingly collected. What more natural than that, while working closely with Mrs. Guthrie, at East Haddon Hall Hospital, Founder in 1910, of the Northamptonshire Hospitals Ladies Linen League[1] and who could drum up support from National and County Nursing Superintendents, he should mention Long Buckby's lack of a nurse. Within 16 months of a public meeting supported by Mrs. Guthrie we had a nurse.

In the modern phraseology "he made things happen".

To go down the other 'side' as it were, it is not certain when Henry Scrase came to the parish. He trained at The London Hospital and qualified L.S.A. and M.R.C.S. in 1830. Pigot's London & Provincial New Commercial Directory, 1830, unfortunately only lists the Dix and Bull practice, so we do not know for certain whom he joined or displaced. Pigot's Directory 1840, first lists him. He was, however, known to be here in 1839 by his inclusion among those serving on Long Buckby Vestry. Qualifying in 1830 it is likely that he came in the early or mid thirties. Directories of 1841 and 1847 show him in single-handed practice. Little is known of him. He was renting a house, buildings and land (5a-0-38p) in 1841 belonging to Mary Wadsworth (Rates Book for the Parish, property of Mrs. Fredrick Buswell).[2] The rateable value was £19-10s-6d and, at the rate of 15d in the pound, his rates were £1-4s-5d. We are able to identify this house by the lucky finding of an amusing receipt which had slipped down the back of the mantel shelf and was found over a century later when alterations to a fireplace in Holly House, High Street, were being made.[3]

References:-

1. Plaque that was on the wall of the inner hall of Northampton General Hospital.
   To the memory of Mary Guthrie of East Haddon, who in the year 1910 founded the Northampton Ladies Linen League in connection with the Northampton General Hospital.
2. An assessment for the Necessary Relief of the Poor and for the other purposes in the several Acts of Parliament etc., 21st April 1841 being the first rate at 15d in the pound in the present year of 1841. Wm Dix owned his house, buildings and 12a 2r 7p of land. House rateable value = £22-16s-0d, land = £8-0s-7d. Total rates at 15d in the pound = £2-13s-4¾d less than the windmill rates at 1s-0½d in the pound and totalling £9-0s-0d.
3. Auther's note – Holly House was a doctor's house for about 100 years.

The 1850 Medical Directory lists Scrase of Northampton.

In the 1847 Medical Directory William Watson is registered of Lutterworth, M.R.C.S., 1843, L.S.A., 1844, formerly M.O., Barrow-on Soar Union. (i.e. Poor Law M.O., in Leicestershire).

The 1848 Medical Directory lists him of Long Buckby. He came between the publication of Kelly's 1847 Directory and Whellan's 1849 Directory which lists Scrase and Watson. So his arrival is double checked. Scrase retired between 1849 and the 1851 Census (2 principals, Dix and Watson – a batchelor – listed). His departure is double checked by the 1850 Medical Directory entry of Northampton.

Watson married Elizabeth Ivens, of the Parish of Long Buckby, on 24th October 1854. Watson's father was described as a farmer and grazier in the Register. Elizabeth Iven's father was described as Yeoman, farmer and grazier. In the 1851 Census he farmed the second largest acreage in the parish, a farm called 'Watson's' (250 acres). Not surprisingly Wm. Watson retired in 1858 in consequence of ill health "and a change in my circumstances enabling me to engage in other pursuits".[1] Whether he inherited land from his father I do not know but he certainly varied the pattern. Instead of investing in land and property he married it. Later, however, he was to own land.

He was described in the 1874 Kelly's Directory of Northamptonshire as farmer and grazier.

The tradition of son following father into the medical profession was continued in this family. William, born 18th February 1861 became a surgeon and practised at Wellingborough.

Although Watson Senior only practised in all for 15 years he worked exceedingly hard in his first year or two here. His entry in the 1848 Medical Directory makes this plain: "Surgeon to Warwick Union and M.O., Daventry Union District No. 4.". The Warwick Union means the Workhouse at Warwick. What a fantastic distance he had to ride at regular intervals in addition to getting about No. 4 District Daventry Union seeing patients. The apothecaries in those days – at least when they were younger – must have kept very fit. Vitually lived in the saddle you might say.

Wm. Watson senior died in 1893.

Arthur Cox born in 1834, the son of a prosperous draper in Market Harborough, grandson of a parson, came to Long Buckby in 1858 and died aged 74 in 1909.

Reference:

1. Letter W. Watson to A. Cox dated 5th August 1858.

Long Buckby, Dec. 22nd, 1858.

Sir,

As the appointment of Medical Officer to the No. 4 District of the Daventry Union, has become vacant by the resignation of Mr. WATSON, I beg to offer myself as a Candidate at the coming election, and request the favour of your Vote and Support.

I am,

Sir,

Yours respectfully,

ARTHUR COX.

*** *Enclosed are copies of my Testimonials, the originals, with the Diplomas, will be forwarded to Mr. Norman.*

Letter from Dr. Arthur Cox applying for post of Medical Officer of Health.

He was apprenticed, aged 15, to Richard Rodd Robinson of Speenhamland in the County of Berks. Surgeon Apothecary and Accoucheur ..."to learn the Art, Science and Profession of a Surgeon, Apothecary and Accoucheur...to serve from the day of the date of these presents (5th September 1849) unto the full end and term of five years...And the said Richard Rodd Robinson for the consideration of the sum of One Hundred and fifty pounds of lawful British money to him in hand...shall and will teach and interest or cause to be taught and instructed finding unto the said apprentice good and sufficient meat drink board and lodging during the first three years of the said term".[1]

Of course there was a lot more. "He shall neither buy nor sell without his said master's licence, Taverns and Inns or Alehouses he shall not haunt, at Cards Dice Tables or any other Unlawful Games he shall not play nor from the service of his said Master day or night unlawfully absent himself".[1]

The interesting thing about this apprenticship Indenture is the stipulation that the apprentice reside in London for two of the five years in order to attend the Hospital and Lectures there. (Hospital not specified but it was King's College Hospital where his son Ernest was also trained). The date of the Indenture was 1849. I do not know whether, by this date, it was the accepted thing for the last two years of the Apprenticeship to be spent in London and, if so, when this became common practice. As University College, London, had been founded in 1826.[2] I should imagine that it was becoming accepted for two of the five years to be spent in hospital, though probably not obligatory as yet. And training by apprenticeship went on. If my surmise is incorrect then Arthur Cox had a very enlightened Master..."And it is hereby agreed between the parties hereto that the said Arthur Cox shall during the last two years of the said term at his own expense or at the expense of the said Thomas Cox (father) his executors or administrators reside in London in order that he may attend the Hospital and Lectures there...And that he the said Thomas Cox shall and will during all the said term of five years find and provide for the said Arthur Cox proper and suitable clothes wearing apparel and linen and the washing and mending thereof and also shall and will during the last two years of the said term of five years find shall and will keep indemnified the said Richard Rodd Robinson his executors administrators and assigns against the same and every part thereof."[3]

References:

1. Mr. Arthur Cox (with the consent of his father Thomas Cox Esq) to Mr. Richard Rodd Robinson Apprenticeship Indenture, 5th September 1849.
2. University of Durham founded in 1832. Medical School, Newcastle upon Tyne opened 1834.
3. Ibid, 1849.

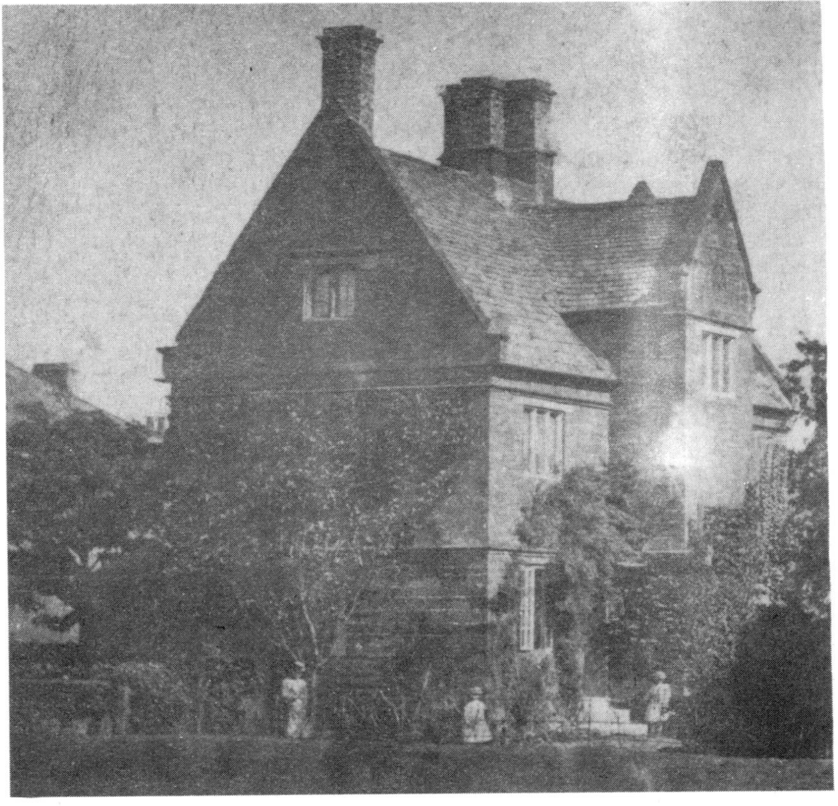

Holly House – Dr. Cox's house – about 1870

So father had a lot more expense than the bare Apprenticeship consideration of £150. Arthur Cox was listed M.R.C.S., L.S.A., 1855.

The practice receipts – £400 approx p.a., £160 of which were from Union and Club appointments – prospects and terms (£200 to be paid down) were satisfactory and Dr. Cox began work in Long Buckby, aged 24, in 1858. William Watson was at pains to point out that the rent of the house (Holly House) with a large garden and paddock was £25 a year.

Watson was prepared, for the £200 down, to give two months introduction and to render his successor much assistance after the expiration of that term.

The house was later purchased for £500. That Watson never owned Holly House is proved by:-

> On Tuesday, June 18th 1850. At the Horse-Shoe Inn, Long Buckby.
> All that capital Stone-built genteel Family freehold Dwelling House.
> Comprising:- 2 Parlours, 4 bedrooms, kitchen and the usual domestic offices, in excellent repair; Surgery with Rooms over, flower and kitchen gardens, Paddock, Yard, Pump of good water, Coach House, Stable, Barn and other appurtenancies thereto adjoining, eligibly situated in the best part of Long Buckby having an entrance from High Street and also an extensive frontage to Meeting Lane, with two entrances therefrom. Also that capital close of land near to the above, 4 acres of good turf; the whole being in the occupation of W. Watson, Esq., Surgeon. Etc.
> Sale to commence at Six O'Clock in the Evening to a minute.

Qualifying in 1855 Arthur Cox must have been the last generation of doctors trained, wholly or in part, by apprenticeship. He began practising in Long Buckby in 1858, the year of the Medical Act, which received the Royal Assent in that year after no fewer than 17 Medical Bills had foundered between 1840 and 1858. The reason for 17 successive Bills being thrown out was conflict of interests or views. By this Act the General Medical Council was set up to supervise medical education and examinations, compile a Register of the medical profession, keep a watch on the ethics and morals of the profession and to publish a national Pharmacopoeia.[1]

Reference:

1. Centenary of the General Medical Council 1858-1958. The History and Present Work of the Council by Walter Pyke-Lees (Registrar of the Council).

In 1875 Cox was listed as District Medical Officer to No.4. District Daventry Union and – beginnings of industrial medicine here – Surgeon to the Railway Friendly Society at Crick and Kilsby Stations, L.N.W. Railway. He was also very well in with the United Brothers' Friendly Society which invited him to the Members' dinner on Whit-Wednesday 1879, at the Admiral Rodney Inn before the General Meeting at 3.0 pm. The chair was taken by the President who was supported by W. Watson (Cox's predecessor, who had obviosly not given up matters medical entirely) by A. Cox and the 'club officers'.[1]

Watson's estimate in his letter to Cox about the practice was that Union (i.e. Poor Law) and Club (Friendly Societies) amounted to about £160 p.a., which represented 40% of his total income. That was in 1858. In 1875 and 1879, after 17 to 21 years of hard work, and becoming very popular, that amount might have substantially and proportionately increased. And the L.N.W.R., was yet to open its loop line from Northampton to Rugby with stations at Long Buckby and Althorp Park providing more potential members of the Railway Friendly Society. The railway in those days was very labour-intensive. This was a time of mutual improvement and self-help in Long Buckby and 2 more Friendly Societies (Star of Hope Benefit Society 1883, and the United Effort Benefit Society, 1884), were to be formed.[2]

True to tradition two of his sons followed him into the profession – Ernest Alfred who entered the practice and Henry Proctor who emigrated to Canada.

References:

1. *Northampton Mercury* 7th June 1879, p.2 col. 6. By Courtesy of Mr.R. Greenall, W.E.A., Long Buckby. 1988.
2. R. Greenall's W.E.A., Lecture, Long Buckby, 1988 'Mutual Improvement and Working People After 1848 in Long Buckby.

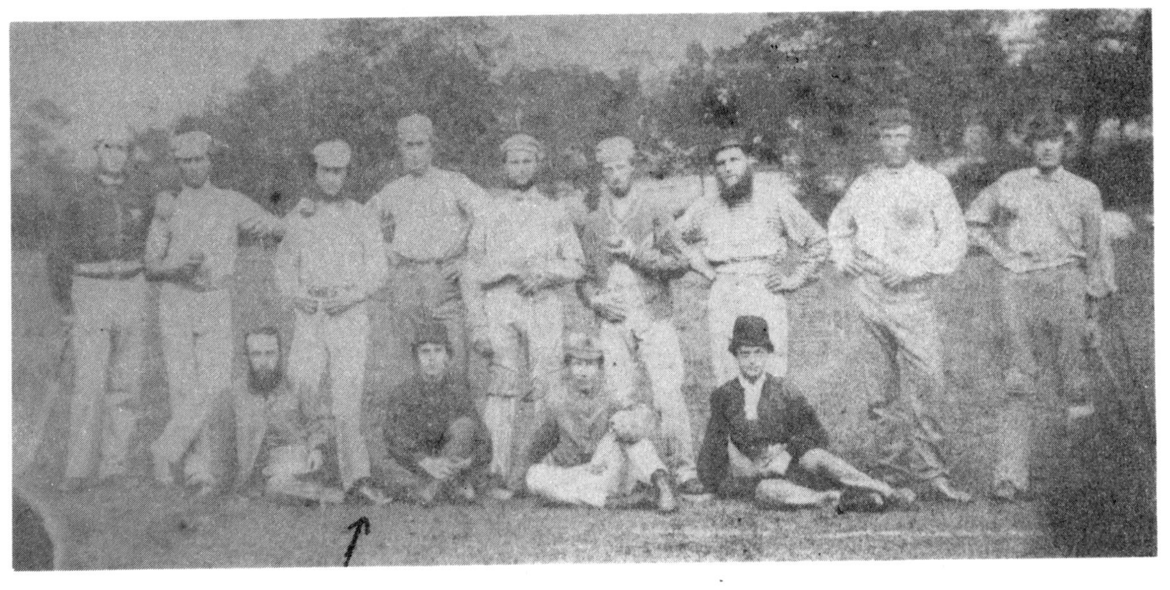

Long Buckby Cricket Team in 1866
Dr. Arthur Cox, then aged 30 – arrowed.

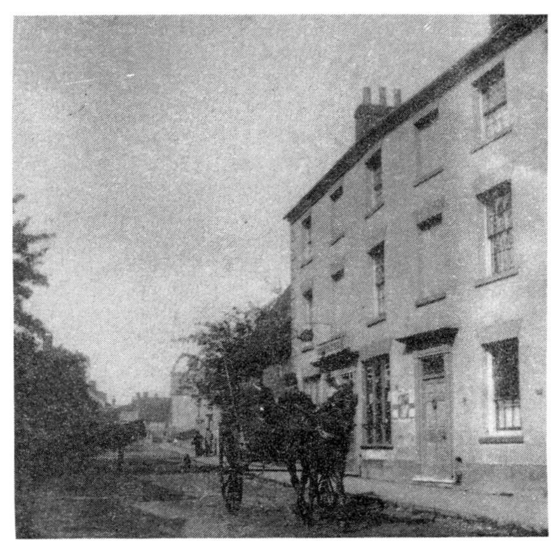

Dr. Cox and coachman, Matthews, in Long Buckby High Street, 1869.

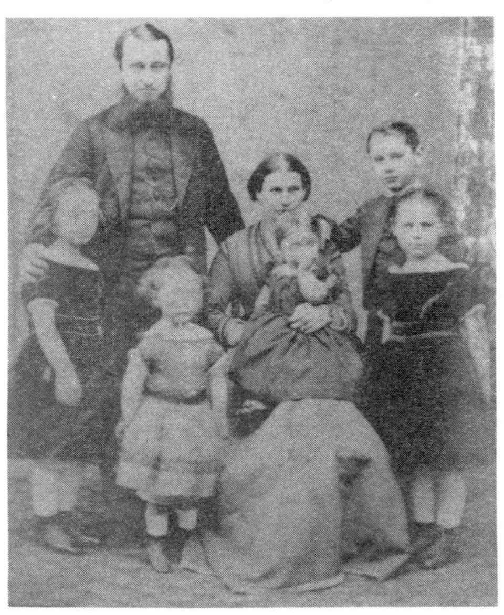

Dr. and Mrs. Arthur Cox with their young family.

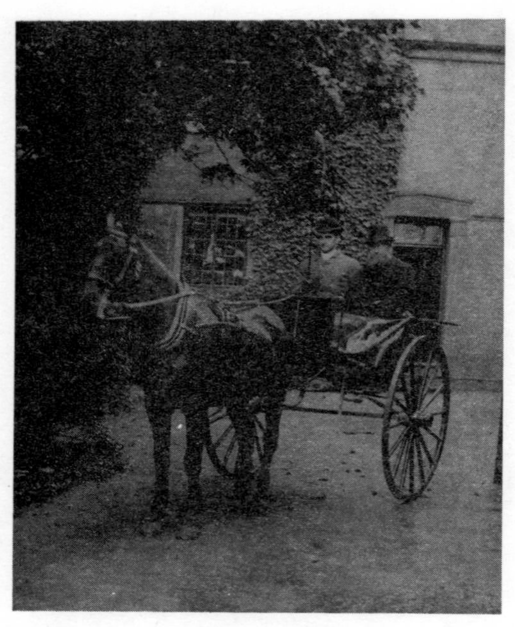

Dr. Cox and Matthews, the coachman, starting on his rounds,1896.

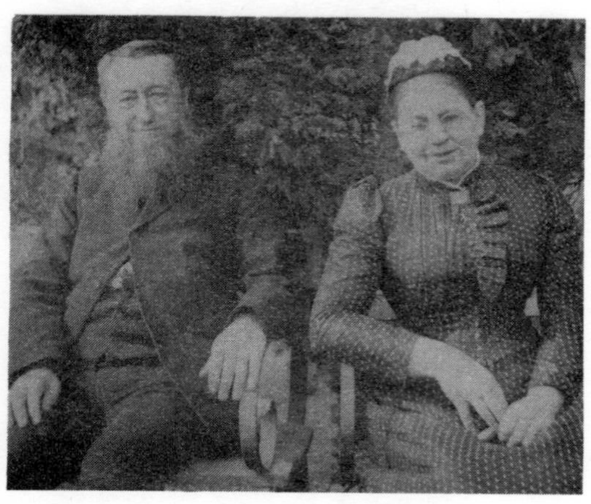

Dr. and Mrs. Arthur Cox in 1892 when he was probably 62.

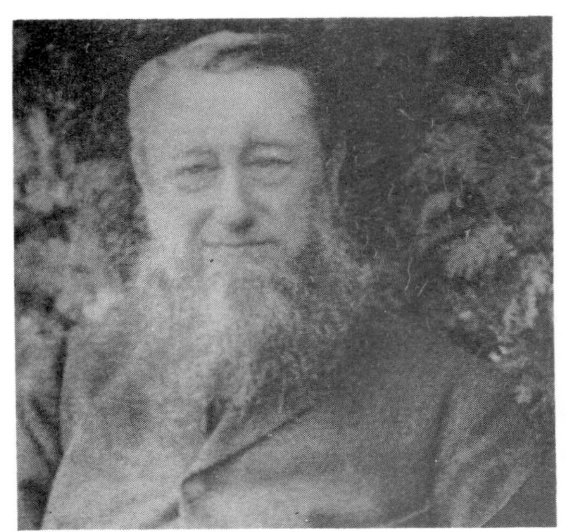

Dr. Arthur Cox, aged 62.

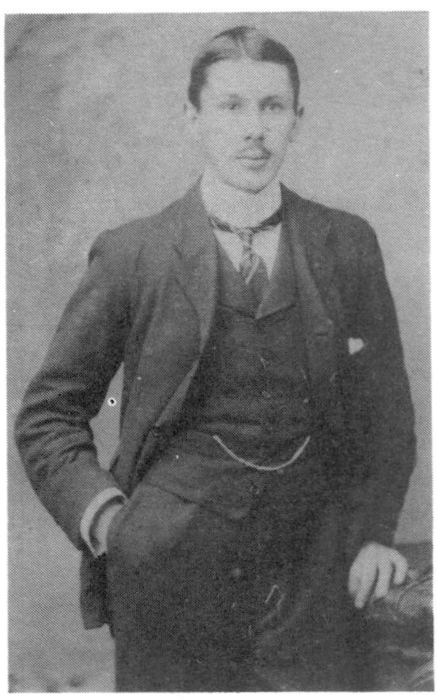

Dr. Ernest Cox about 1896.

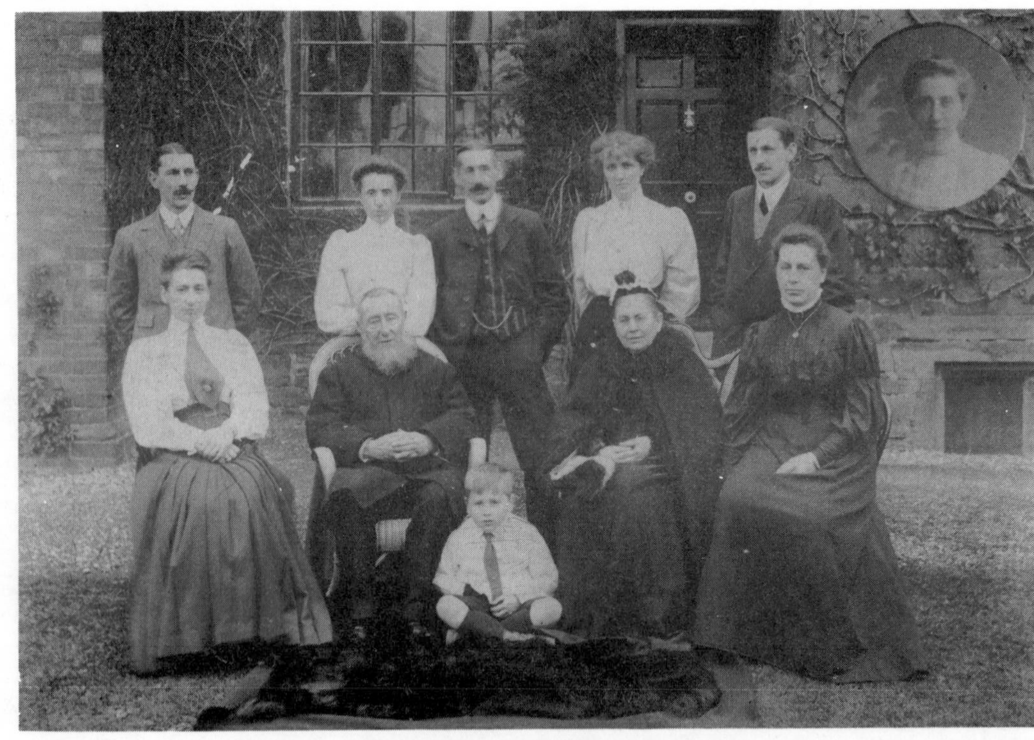

Dr. Arthur Cox and family in 1908.

3. The Impact of Infection and and Communicable Disease

It is difficult for those born before preventive medicine really got under way to remember, and well nigh impossible for those born in the vaccine-for-everything era and antibiotic age to imagine, what it was like before there was effective treatment for most illnesses and the severe effect some Infectious Diseases could have on the community.

Scarlet Fever was being talked of as a changed disease in the last 30 years in the late 1930s and 1940s. No longer the scourge it was; no longer the serious illness with profound toxaemia and severe complications, it could still disrupt education for 9 months in the Junior School. "1929 March – Our attendance has been poor right along from the Summer Holiday owing to a prolonged epidemic of Scarlet Fever and Diptheria, but the last week or two with 8° of frost a sharp attack of colds, influenza, chicken pox, more scarlet fever and diptheria has reduced us this week to 74.7% attendance." [1]

We read...1913 February "Re-opened school after a holiday of 6 weeks owing to an epidemic of measles."

Late last century, but for the kindness of Bishop Mitchinson, scarlet fever would have been responsible for our Candidates missing their Confirmation.

"Confirmation — owing to the prevalence of scarlet fever in Long Buckby, it was thought inadvisable that our Candidates should be presented for Confirmation at West Haddon as was originally intended. Bishop Mitchinson, therefore, very kindly, after administering the Sacred Rite at Blisworth in the morning, and at West Haddon in the afternoon of May 7th, came to our Parish Church at 5.0 p.m., on the same day. The arrangements were only altered at the last moment and our thanks"[2]...etc. etc.

The Bishop had a long day but the decision was absolutely right in the circumstances as a 'Carrier' amongst our Candidates or their families would undoubtedly have spread the disease to West Haddon. And West Haddon would have been decidedly displeased.

References:

1. Junior School Log Books.
2. Long Buckby Church Monthly Magazine, June 1896.

Acute infectious disease could cause heartrending suffering to parents. Two months before the only surviving child was accidentally shot and killed, her brother and sister, aged 2 and 6 years respectively, had died of diphtheria.[1] Prior to this there were 26 cases of diphtheria in 1892 and 1893 resulting in 6 deaths.

From the Notes (Editorial) – Long Buckby Parish Magazine October 1887 we read "The following is an extract from a Sermon which was preached in our Parish Church on September 20th 1885. It had reference to the Cholera which was then raging on the Continent; but the drift of the remarks applied equally to the Typhoid Fever which has attacked nearly 60 persons in our Parish during this summer, and is still busy. Thank God that it has not reached England, as many feared it would. It may do so another year; who can tell? But remember this: whether we are able to stamp it out quickly, or whether it will decimate our land as it has done others, will depend in great measure upon the food which it finds ready for its support and the nourishment which we, with reckless generosity, lay in its way. Don't think that God will listen to our prayers for help when the remedy is in our own hands; when foul drains, filthy cesspools and polluted water abound in our midst. If the Cholera comes, there is the food that it loves ready spread out for its reception, as it were a welcome guest. Thank God then all the more that it has not come".[2]
(Rev. A. Oswel James).

Whether he preached too soon and Cholera reached England I do not know. I can find no record of its striking Long Buckby.

There had been an outbreak of Cholera (about 70 cases with 19 deaths) in Braunston, 6 miles away, in the autumn of 1834 brought by a boatman on the Grand Junction Canal. The Registrar-General, Report on Cholera in England, 1848-49 gave Long Buckby, Pop. 5613 – Cholera 1; Diarrhoea 2. He was a labourer's son aged 2, after an attach of 24 hours duration. He presumably died.

But what a way of celebrating Queen Victoria's Golden Jubilee! Sixty seven cases in all of Typhoid were recorded and a further five cases occurred in 1890. The doctors must have derived considerable clinical experience of the disease and become local authorities on it.

Strong words from the vicar; and his eloquent preaching combined with a pracatical and temporal approach may not have made him very popular at a time when hygiene and sanitation were not considered very important. And Dr. Franklin Churchouse, as Medical Officer to the local Board of Health and Rural Sanitary District, was making no headway in popularising his views on Long Buckby's sanitation.

Back on a personal level and demonstrating the devastating effect that communicable disease could have on people there is a report of a Concert given by the Band. This was highly successful and was in aid of Mr. Thomas Amos (a member of the choir), eight of whose family had contracted the disease.

References:

1. Long Buckby Church Monthly Magazine April 1900.
2. Long Buckby Parish Magazine October 1887.

No Amos names appeared in the Anglican Burial Registers for the three years. Complications would have been another matter and it might well have been that two or three – or more Amoses suffered from the less life-endangering complications of Typhoid.

The Vicar got in his bit again. "We hope the prevalence of this epidemic will make us all more careful about the state of our drains and the quality of our water. What else but fever can we expect when the sewerage runs into the well! It is lamentable to think that much sickness might have been averted if more prompt attention had been paid to the unsatisfactory condition of many of our dwelling houses."[1]

Smallpox, while perhaps not rife, could occur at any time – Vestry minutes noted cases in 1834 – so it is impossible to say, as the 19th Century wore on, whether the doctors appointed by the Vestry of the Parish Church to attend the poor, their duties to include Midwifery, Small Pox (sic) and accidents, were reducing the incidence of smallpox locally. The inclusion of smallpox in their medical duties may have meant, of course, attendance of cases rather than vaccination. This provision was first noted in 1832.

As the Vaccination Act 1898 received the Royal Assent on the 12th August of that year it is reasonable to suppose that the national incidence was not dropping.

As devoted to public health, and dedicated to preventive medicine as were the Medical Officers of Health and Vaccination Officers in the Poor Law Union and, no doubt other colleagues, the doctors did not, however, have it all their own way. You could become a card-carrrying member of the Long Buckby and District Anti-Compulsory Vaccination Society, minimum weekly subscription 1d paid monthly, with 6d entrance fee. Rule 2 states – That the objects of the Society shall be (a) to take any action that may be deemed advisable to promote the total repeal of the Compulsory Vaccination Acts (there must have been earlier ones); and (b) to assist, by paying their fine and costs as far as the funds will allow, those members who may be prosecuted for non-compliance with the Acts; (c) in cases where members are willing to allow distraint instead of paying fines, to render assistance upon the same conditions. Rule 6 states – That when a member is summoned or otherwise proceeded against he shall immediately inform the Secretary. Any person who is not a member but has received a summons can only be admitted on payment of a fee of 5s.[2]

References:

1. Long Buckby Parish Magazine November 1887.
2. Membership Card of Long Buckby and District Anti-Compulsory Vaccination Society 1897-8.

Strong Stuff. I wonder if any cases of refusal, or inability, to pay the fine ever went so far as levying distraint[1] upon the person, or whether the process usually stopped at distraint upon his goods in order to meet the fine.

So were the Anti-Compulsory Vaccination Society and the refusal of most of the villagers to realise how bad the water supply was and how appalling the sanitation, examples of sturdy independence of mind or downright ignorant conservatism? With nearly a century of hindsight it is easy for us to answer that question.

The existence of an organized body of opposition to preventive medicine 100 years after Jennerian vaccination was first introduced following publication of Jenner's investigations in 1798, contrasts strongly with the state of affairs in the remote rural community of Guilsborough. This was in the forefront of the times as regards health and education. There, inoculation for smallpox was practised as early as 1761 when we find the village doctor offering to treat "gentlemen and others"..."after the best manner at reasonable rates" (i.e. introduction into the system of the smallpox virus from a mild case).

Advertisements in the Northampton Mercury, November 1761. "All Gentlemen and Others, that are disposed to be inoculated for Small Pox (sic) may apply to Robert Goodman in Nortoft Grounds in the Parish of Guilsborough, Northamptonshire; where they may, by the Assistance of an Apothecary, be inoculated and Nursed after the best manner at reasonable Rates. Any Surgeon, Doctor or Apothecary, who please to recommend any Person or Persons, may be sure of finding very good Receptions, upon reasonable terms from:

Their Humble Servant,
Robert Goodman".[2]

In 1771 Goodman's terms were "Two Pounds Eight Shillings, being the whole expense, wine only excepted – Patients from home at Half-a-Guinea, and Servants at Half Price."

In 1790 he broke into doggerel "Inoculation".

By Robert Goodman, of Guilsborough, at a Lodge in the Parish of Guilsborough, at Two Guineas each Patient for a fortnight, all necessaries (Wine excepted).

References:

1. *Concise Oxford Dictionary, 5th Edition.* Distrain vi (legal) Levy a distress (upon a person or his goods), seize chattels to compel person to pay money due (esp. rent) or to meet an obligation, or to obtain satisfaction by sale of chattels. Hence -er, -ee, -ment distraint, nn.
2. Records of Guilsborough, Nortoft and Hollowell, Northamptonshire. Compiled by Ethel L. Renton and Eleanor L. Renton. 1929.

"All that please for to put themselves under My care./May depend on good Usuage and good proper Fare;/-For twenty odd years, this My business I've made/And thought, by Much People, to well know my Trade./ Then be not in Doubt, but with Speed to me come./ By the Blessing of God, I send you safe Home!".[1]

The last inoculation advertisement in the Mercury was in 1794. [1]

I wonder if the Long Buckby apothecaries referred patients.

All the foregoing cannot be compared to rabies for drama.

"News of two of our boys and a Watford (village) man bitten by a mad dog was followed by the Doctors and Our County Councillor promptly telegraphing the Mansion House in London requesting an immediate grant from the Lord Mayor's Special Fund. Within 24 hours of the receipt of his telegram promising a contribution of £15 towards the expenses of sending the three sufferers to Paris, they were actually under treatment at the Pasteur Institute with the first ever human vaccine discovered by Louis Pasteur."[2]

Pasteur's account of his rabies discoveries in 1885 produced a profound impression. Patients arrived from all parts of France and the world. Nineteen Russian peasants, terribly bitten by a rabid wolf, arrived from Smolensk. Four children came from New York, their travelling expenses paid by an American newspaper. An English policeman, a Basque peasant, and many others could be seen at the laboratory which must, at times, have more resembled a hospital outpatients' than a research institute.

Speed was the essence of the operation. The incubation period could be as short as ten days if the patient was extensively bitten or badly bitten about the head, and, once symptoms of rabies developed, death was inevitable in dog or man.

Our 'patients' probably had a good prognosis but, unfortunately, there was no further reference to the matter.

Not so a later case. The Long Buckby Church Monthly Magazine September 1890 reports:-

"Rabies. We have had to send another of our Parishioners (the third within twelve months) to Paris to be treated at the Pasteur Institute. In this case there was a regrettably long interval of 4-5 weeks between the bite and the lad's departure." (average incubation period 50-60 days *R.G.L.)*.

References:

1. As reference 2, previous page.
2. Long Buckby Church Monthly Magazine, November 1889.

"The dog which bit him escaped and there was no proof of its condition until another dog which it had also bitten, died of rabies; then no time was lost in making the medical arrangements. The Lord Mayor again gave a liberal contribution from his Fund; and for the rest, an account has been opened at the Union Bank where contributions will be received, by kind permission of Mr. Bunting, from any who desire to assist."

The Muzzling Order was then criticised. It was said that the mad dog that visited us was muzzled.

Ends "Every care should be taken by owners of dogs to provide them with suitable muzzles and it is worthy of consideration that those which afford the best protection to ourselves are the least irritating to our canine friends."[1]

At least there was no Anti-Inoculation-against-Rabies-Society!

Reference:

1. Long Buckby Church Monthly Magazine, September 1890.

4. Doctors taking part in Local Affairs

This is the story of two doctors. One, the most popular doctor Long Buckby has ever had; the other, at one time, the most unpopular man in the village.

More than 650 of his patients subscribed to Dr. Arthur Cox's testimonial in 1891. It was not his Silver Wedding; nor did the occasion represent 25 years in practice. Neither was it his Golden Wedding nor was he retiring – it was a spontaneous expression of esteem and gratitude. That he was highly revered is made clear by the Church Monthly Magazine, as evidenced by the following. For no reason other than that he had practised for 32 years it reported a "Presentation to Mr. Cox. An illuminated address and cheque for 20 guineas and a medical work in 2 volumes. A token of esteem in grateful recognition of his unvarying kindness and attention to his professional duties during a period of 32 years."[1]

One feels he epitomized 'The Doctor' in Sir Luke Fildes's world famous picture, now hanging in the Tate Gallery, which became the most popular print the firm of Agnew's ever issued.

Dr. Franklin Churchouse owed his unpopularity, in part, to his attempts to get the use of the market place as a camp site at the 'Feast' stopped. "At the annual village festival or feast there encamp in the market square around one of the public pumps a considerable number of travelling show folk with their vans and caravans. On medical testimony it is stated that these people befoul the surface of the ground with slop water, urine and excrement, which in wet weather, it has been urged, might easily be washed through the porous soil and ultimately reach the well. The late Medical Office of Health, recognising this evident danger, took steps to get the market place as a camping place stopped; but his efforts were defeated by the villagers themselves who, with misdirected sympathy, espoused the cause of the nomadic show people, with the result that this danger still occurs year by year when 'the feast' comes round."[2]

Arthur Cox was elected to the first Parish Council on December 17th 1894 and, in April 1895, was appointed to serve on the Sanitary Committee. He did not seek re-election at the second Parish Election, on the 9th March 1896. Nor did he become Medical Officer of Health to the Daventry Rural District after Franklin Churchouse. Dr. Darley of West Haddon took over.

References:

1. Long Buckby Church Magazine April 1891.
2. Dr. Bruce Low's report to the Local Government Board on the Water Supply of Long Buckby in the Rural District of Daventry, Northants. November 26th 1896.

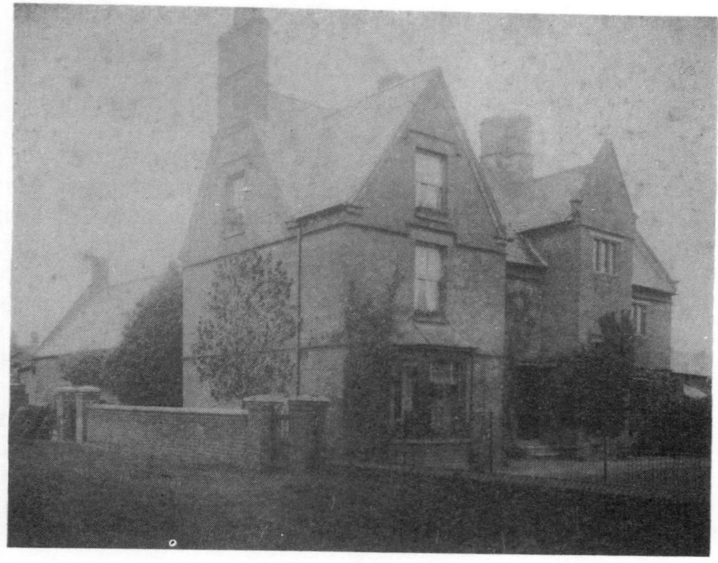

Holly House, Dr. Cox's house about 1900 with brick wing added.

No; Arthur Cox's interest outside medicine was the church. From his obituary – "Dr. Cox settled in the town in September 1858 and took a keen interest in its welfare, especially in the affairs of the church, where he regularly attended services. He filled the office of Churchwarden in the years 1867-8 and again in 1874 until Easter 1887; but previous to this took an active part in the first restoration of the church in 1862-3 by serving on the committee whose many meetings he generally attended. He was Churchwarden during the onerous times of the restoration of the aisles in 1882-3 and 1886-7. He also took part in the ministrations of the church by conducting for some time the services at Buckby Wharf...etc".[1]

He was a Director of Long Buckby Gas Co. Truly a giant of the past.

What can be said of a doctor who failed to be elected to the first Parish council in 1894 by the ignominiously lowest poll and who was sacked from his appointment as Medical Officer of Health? Paragraph 2 of the Summary of Dr. R. Bruce Low's Report reads "These well waters have been condemned repeatedly on sanitary grounds by the late Medical Officer of Health who lost his appointment recently as a result of his insisting upon the need for a new supply...etc".[2]

Franklin Churchouse was M.o.H., for 10 years – first to the local Board of Health and Rural Sanitary District, later to the Daventry Rural District Council.

He was a zealot. And who really likes a zealot!?

But it was his single-minded determination, his dogged perseverance and his uncompromising views on all matters concerning Long Buckby's hygiene, sanitation and water supply that mark him out. In the years 1887 to 1895 Dr. Churchouse, as M.o.H., repeatedly drew the attention of the Daventry Board of Health to the connection between Typhoid Fever in Long Buckby and its polluted well water.

"In 1891 and again in 1894 professional experts were engaged by the local authority to inquire into the subject. The result of these inquiries confirmed Dr. Churchouse's statements. Nevertheless no definite steps were taken to provide a better water supply for Long Buckby. Dr. Churchouse's action in condemning the wells in the village created considerable feeling against him among the local representatives on the

Rural District Council of Daventry, and when the re-election of this officer came up for discussion in December 1895, he failed to secure re-appointment...".[2]

References:

1. Long Buckby Church Magazine March 1909.

2. Dr. R. Bruce Low's Report, 1896.

It was openly mentioned in the local press that the R.D.C. had no fault to find with Dr. Churchouse as regarded the discharge of his duties during the ten years he had been their Medical Officer of Health, but that his continued insistence upon the necessity for providing a fresh water supply for Long Buckby had given serious offence to the councillors, and that his failure to secure re-election was the punishment meted out to him for his pertinacity."[1]

An interesting state of affairs arose about this time of one doctor wanting to get off the Parish Council and one wanting to get on. Arthur Cox did not become a candidate at the second Parish Council election on 9th March. He could see the way things were going and was not risking certain controversy and possible obloquy. Franklin Churchouse had to wait for election until 1898. Having recently lost his appointment as M.o.H., he must have hoped to further his cause by becoming an insider. Did Arthur Cox apply for the M.o.H., appointment in December 1895 and was not selected or did he not apply? Almost certainly the latter in view of his not wishing to stand again for the P.C.

To give an idea how bad the sanitation and water supply of the place were, and what Franklin Churchouse was so vehement about, one cannot do better than quote Dr. Low's report. "The village is not sewered. For a number of years slop water has been discharged into the square highway drains which are imperfectly constructed...Excrement is disposed of mainly by vault or cesspit privies situated in back yards, and emptied usually at long intervals by the occupiers on fields, allotments or gardens...Some cesspits were seen overflowing upon the surface of yards. There are a few (less than a dozen) water closets in the place...Refuse is disposed of in open ashpits or in middens in back yards...The ashpits and middens are emptied sometimes twice a year by the occupiers, some that I saw had not been emptied for nearly two years...In emptying ashpits and middens it is usual to throw the contents out upon the surface of the garden or yard, sometimes even upon the street, then with spade and bucket to empty the excrement from the cesspit or privy-pit upon the heap and finally to mix the whole together before it is carted way to agricultural land, or spread upon allotments or gardens...A large number of occupiers keep pigs in their back yards. Many of these animals are kept too near dwellings, the sty is often wet creating a nuisance.

"Long Buckby derives its water supply from about 116 local wells, some six of which are public...the majority of the wells are dry steined (sic) – (presumably meaning unmortared stone walled) and many are not protected from the direct entrance of storm water nor from lateral soakage into them of liquid filth...the appearance of many samples of water shown to me during the inspection was bright and clear, but many of the wells from which the samples in question were taken had been condemned by chemical analysis...the highway drains are in places merely open fronted square culverts permitting escape of their liquid contents into the soil, and, as some wells are situated in the streets, contamination of the water from this source is probable."

Reference:

1. Dr. R.Bruce Low's Report 1896.

It is difficult a century later to comprehend the technical distinctions between vault and cesspit privies; ashpits and middens; and to understand the finer points of disposal. What seems certain is that there was no shortage of manure in Long Buckby even though the distribution from the points of production was tardy.

In 1895 the Local Government Board (i.e. Whitehall) was pressing the Parish Council for a new water supply and sewerage for Long Buckby. The P.C. replied "that it was doing all in its power to protect the water supply from contamination by laying down glazed, socketed pipes wherever required...And by frequent inspection of all privies and cesspools...They also wish to draw attention to the Medical Officer's report for 1895 which compares very favourably with any previous report sent in by him and tends to prove that the efforts used have been eminently successful."[1]

Conditions were no different so, because no typhoid fever had been reported and other infectious disease (presumably) was less, the P.C. inferred that the Medical Officer's report compared favourably with others. The L.G.B. obviously did not agree. A month later, 19th August 1895, a letter from the L.G.B. drew attention to the Medical Officer's report and pressed for urgent action on a new water and sewarage system.[2]

So the P.C. called for the Medical Officer's reports for 1893, 1894 and 1895!

4th September 1895 – The Medical Officer's reports for 1893, '94, '95, having been considered, it was proposed and seconded "that the Council is of the opinion that the Medical Officer's report for 1895 does not point to any serious defect of the water supply..." etc. Carried 12 to 1.[3]

References:

1. Long Buckby Parish Council Minutes – early years.
2. Ibid, 19th August 1895.
3. Ibid, 4th September 1895.

Who was the lone and enlightened dissentient? However, the P.C. decided that the Sanitary Committee of the Council obtain samples of water from 12 different wells in the town for analysis. These 2 resolutions were sent to the Rural Sanitary Authority.[1] In the event only 6 samples were sent to the analyst on account of the expense.

On 30th September 1895 the M.o.H. wrote directly to the P.C. The minutes state grave statements about the water supply were made.[2] Obviously there was a serious difference of opinion on the quality of the water supply between the Long Buckby P.C. on the one hand and the M.o.H., (still Franklin Churchouse) and the L.G.B., on the other.

The P.C. had a nasty shock on 11th October 1895.

Professor Attfield's report begins: "The Appended Analytical data enable me to give the opinion that the whole of these 6 samples of water are badly contaminated by Animal or Vegetable and Mineral Matter and that not one of them is fit to be used for drinking purposes...Warrants me in condemning the whole subsoil supply from which the wells have enabled the 6 samples to be drawn...I cannot regard any of the 6 samples as fairly indicating the normal uncontaminated water supply of the district...All that I can at present say is that the contamination has all the characters of ordinary sewerage contamination."[3]

As if the general report were not bad enough, at the bottom of the Organic Analysis of the 6 Long Buckby samples:

Nos.	1	2	3	4	5	6
Potable Quality	Bad	Bad	Bad	Bad	Bad	Bad

So the P.C., had no option but to propose and second (Prop. Dr. Cox, Sec. W. Haynes), but only after considerable discussion, "that, after hearing Professor Attfield's report, the Council believes that steps should be taken to procure a better water supply."[4]

References:

1. Long Buckby Parish Council Minutes, 4th September 1895.
2. Long Buckby Parish Council Minutes 30th September 1895.
3. Copy of Analysis by Professor Attfield, 17 Bloomsbury Sq., London. W.C., 10th October 1895.
4. Long Buckby Parish Council Minutes, 11th October 1895.

However, the P.C. felt that no steps could be taken before a Parish Meeting was called. At this meeting, with the evidence of the report on the 6 samples of well water, a resolution that the Parish take no steps to procure a new water supply was proposed and seconded and even supported by 8 people.[1]

The new P.C. elected in March 1896, was still discussing water at great length and sent 4 more samples for analysis, 3 satisfactory, 1 unfit for drinking. In August yet another 3 samples were analysed and all were reported unfit for drinking. In other circumstances all this chemical analysis would have been right up Franklin Churchouse's street. His obituary stated he was Demonstrator in chemistry at Charing Cross Hospital and Medical School.[2] As it was it must have driven him nearly to distraction. He knew all this as he had induced the Rural Authority to have water specimens analysed in 1891 (Eunson, Engineer, Northampton Waterworks), April 1893 (Fisher, Public Analyst, Oxon., Berks. and Bucks.) and July 1893 (Emerson, Public Analyst. Leicester).[3]

At this time Daventry R.D.C. was pressing Long Buckby P.C. about a new water supply for the village. Again after considerable discussion it was proposed and seconded, and carried unanimously, that the P.C. leave the question of a new water supply to the D.C. "At the same time they protest against it as unnecessary and hope, if the D.C. see their way to avert it, they will, if possible, do so."

Words fail the writer!

It seems a prima facie case of ignorance and bigotry, but we shall see.

Franklin Churchouse was elected for the first time to the P.C. on 14th March 1898 and, at its first meeting, the whole council was voted to be the Sanitary Committee.

Actually, despite the P.C.'s stonewalling in council and by calling a Parish Meeting, the D.C. had, the previous year, been getting on with matters. After Dr. Bruce Low's report had been received, a special committee resolved to advertise for schemes for a water supply and offered a premium of 30 guineas for the best scheme. Out of 17 sets of plans received the Long Buckby Water Committee chose one costing £3,470 and recommended to the D.C. that a trial boring for water at an estimated cost of £350 be made.

References:

1. The bare account of this Parish Meeting was included in the Long Buckby Parish Council Minutes 11th October 1895.
2. Obituary – Dr. W.J. Franklin Churchouse, *Northampton Independent,* 10th December 1927.
3. Dr. Bruce Low's Report to the Local Govt. Board on the Water Supply of Long Buckby in the Rural District of Daventry, Northants. 1896.

Boring operations commenced on 8th July 1898 and, by the 3rd September, 163 feet had been reached. Water was eventually found at a depth of 323 feet. All should have been well. Dr. Churchouse had been requested to write to Northampton asking for recommendations for a suitable man as Clerk of the Works.

Discontent with the progress of the preliminary boring was soon being voiced. 2.1.1899 – Motion by Dr. Churchouse Sec. by Mr.P. Webb "that the P.C. is dissatisfied with the progress of the waterworks".[1]

The next month a P.C. motion stated that the P.C. is very dissatisfied with the neglect of the D.C. in not exercising more supervision..."[2] etc. (but the P.C. had been requested in May 1898 to appoint a Clerk of the Works. Was this not done? If it was, was there no accountability?).

All very unsatisfactory, and Franklin Churchouse and Rev. R.A. Parsons (Vicar, a water protagonist) were not re-elected to the P.C. in March 1899.

Later in the year there were open discussions and criticism of the delay and the cost – and this was only the trial boring – and there were fears of the effect on the rates.

While trial boring had been allowed to go on, complications over the purchase of the site of the proposed reservoir had delayed a beginning on the waterworks proper, and this was the state of affairs when Churchouse stepped in again in 1901.

He wrote over the heads of Daventry direct to the County Council: "I cannot think that the County Council realize the responsibility and danger the District Council are incurring in allowing matters to go on as at present, and I propose to bring a few facts to the notice of the County Council in the hope that they may use their influence to induce the District Council to hurry the matter on. I am quite aware what a fatal error was made by the District Council in boring on land without first ascertaining that it could be bought at a reasonable price but surely if in two years they have not been able to agree with the owner as to the terms, it is time to look out a site elsewhere; and as it happens there are three sites, two of which I believe would be available and equally suitable within a few yards of the old site and it seems probable that one of these might be obtained at a reasonable price."[3]

References:

1. Long Buckby Parish Council Minutes 2nd January 1899.
2. Ibid. February 1899.
3. Letter Churchouse to Chairman, The Sanitary Committee, Northampton County Council. 10th August 1901.

He recapitulates the medical details and mentions all the analyses and goes on..."The Daventry Rural District Council are incurring a very serious responsibility in neglecting to provide Long Buckby with a proper Water Supply. On April 20th 1897 the Scheme of Messrs. Usill, Brown and Usill was adopted and two years ago a trial boring was made and a plentiful supply found and there the matter appears to rest; at all events no work has been done during the last ywo years towards providing the Water Supply, and we seem as far off obtaining it now as when I first called attention to it fourteen years ago."[1].

Naturally this would not endear him to Daventry Rural District Council. After a non-committal reply from the County M.o.H., he again wrote to the County Council..."In 1895 I reported the Daventry R.D.C. as a Defaulting Authority to the Local Government Board and the visit of Dr. Bruce Low was the result, I enclose his report...I was hoping the County Council might make a representation of the state of affairs to the Local Government Board as, I believe, they alone have the power to either compel the District Council to get on with the work or step in and do it for them...I thought a letter from the C.C. would have much more effect than one from a private individual. Our representatives on the D.C. consist of two large farmers both residing about a mile and a half out of the village, who will have to pay the rates but will get no possible benefit from the water supply, and the other is a local grocer who owns a great deal of cottage property in the place and is, and always has been, the strongest opponent of the water supply so much so in fact that it was he who proposed that I should not be re-elected as Medical Officer of Health in 1895 so, as you can imagine, none of these men are very keen about pushing on the water supply...Between ourselves, I am afraid nothing will be done by the R.D.C. unless very strong pressure is brought to bear on them from outside and they will take every possible opportunity of putting off what they consider the 'evil day' as long as possible...In the meantime there can, I think, be no doubt of the frightful risk we are running should a case of Enteric (Typhoid) Fever occur at the upper end of the village; how we have escaped since 1890 is a miracle."[2]

That did the trick. On September 17th 1901 the R.D.C. took steps to petition the L.G.B. authorising them to put into force compulsory powers to purchase the land. Then there was delay before the confirmation by Parliament of the Provisional Order prior to arbitration and purchase of the land. The final delay occured when it was found that the proposed works encroached on the 60 foot highway and the boring was re-sited further from the road

References:

1. Letter – Churchouse to Chairman, the Sanitary Committee, Northampton County Council, 10th August 1901.
2. Letter – Churchouse to Dr. Paget, M.o.H., Northampton County Council, 21st August 1901.

Long Buckby Water Supply.

"The provision of a public water supply for Long Buckby is, after many years' delay, an accomplished fact, the water having been turned on to the town last week, although the waste water from the experimental pumping has been used by the inhabitants for the last few weeks. It is principally owing to the untiring efforts of Dr. Churchouse and the late Rev. R.A. Parsons that the works have been carried out..."[1] etc. From recommendation it all took 18 years.

Franklin Churchouse was again to the fore, and took the chair, at a public meeting held with the object of securing a District Nurse for Long Buckby and Whilton.[2] A committee of 20 was elected and the organization was purely voluntary; offers of subscriptions were invited. There were no other references to a District Nurse until September 1902, then in 1904, it was reported that the Long Buckby Self Assistance Industrial Society (the Co-operative Soc.) declined to contribute to the funds of the Long Buckby Nursing Association on the grounds that individual subscriptions had been invited.[3]

At long last another public meeting was held, chaired by the Vicar, supported by Mrs. Guthrie of East Haddon, with a very good attendance. District Nurse for Long Buckby.

> "The provision of a District Nurse for the Parish has been a long-felt want, and it is with pleasure that we report that steps are now being taken to form in Long Buckby a branch of the Northamptonshire County Nursing Association. Mrs. Guthrie of East Haddon, who has always at heart the best interests of our Parish, is now moving in this matter, and we sincerely hope that her efforts may meet with success".[4]

They did. I can sense Franklin Churchouse's influence working behind scenes here. The Long Buckby Church Magazine reported that the District Nurse had been appointed and would be beginning work in October.[5] It was, however, 17 years before Franklin Churchouse's original initiative became reality.

Were this and the duration of the piped water saga not true they would read like an apologue on the virtue of patience.

Dr. W. King Churchouse did not figure in the Minutes as a Member of the Parish Council until after 1929.

In the view of the writer, Franklin Churchouse is quite the most outstanding medical personality Long Buckby has had.

References:

1. *Northampton Herald,* 27th October 1905.
2. Long Buckby Church Monthly Magazine, October 1899.
3. Ibid, August 1904.
4. Ibid, June 1915.
5. Long Buckby Church Magazine, September 1916.

5. Druggists and Pharmacists.

While strictly not medical the chemists took over from the apothecaries as the chief purveyors of medicine and, therfore, deserve their place in any account of medicine.

The interesting things are the diversity of the druggists in the last century and the length of time the present pharmacy has been a chemist's premises.

The Northamptonshire Record Office's Commercial Directories have been invaluable in finding their names. Pigot and Co's London and Provincial New Commercial Directory 1841 gives us our first chemist – Thomas March, while Henry Tilley is described as Chymist and Druggist and John Clark is also listed as Druggist. There may have been earlier chemists and Thomas March may well have been in business before this date had there been an earlier directory to prove it. He was, in fact, listed as an Assessor of the Poor in 1838, and his Assessed Tax for the year ending 5th April 1815, on a 5-windowed house was 6/6d (Collector's Duplicate Book of First Assessments – Mrs. George Thompson's property).

In 1847, Kelly's Directory of Northamptonshire lists John Ringrose – grocer and druggist; John Clarke – grocer, druggist and fellmonger[1] also described as a distributor of stamps, while Thomas March is called a druggist and stationer.

Wm Whellan's General & Manorial History & Directory of Northamptonshire (Mrs. George Thompson's property) 1849 lists Marsh (sic) T. druggist and hairdresser and Driver, John, cooper, drugs and stationery dealer. T. Marsh either felt he was losing trade by not cutting hair or he stepped into the opening left by John Clark (at any rate no longer listed commercially but possibly one and the same as John Clarke listed as grocer and grazier).

The 1864 Post Office Directory of six counties (Mrs. George Thompson's property) lists Mr. March (no occupation).

Chemists Clarke, Thomas M. – grocer, druggist and dealer in foreign and british (sic) wines. March, Thos, Junior – druggist and stationer. So the son had obviously taken over the business and was to advertise in directories until 1877. The 1847 Kelly's Directory of Northamptonshire lists John Clarke, grocer, druggist, fellmonger and distributor of stamps. Slater's Directory of 1862 is more explicit. Clarke, Thomas Marriott is described as grocer, dealer in foreign and British Wines, Post Office.

Herbert Henry Newitt (Associate of the Pharmaceutical Society) arrived in 1879 and first advertised in the January 1884 number of the Long Buckby Parish Magazine (the second one of all) and advertised regularly thereafter. He ran a wool and worsted shop which was also was a general store (stationery, photograph and scrap albums, purses, desks, perfumery, patent medicines, wines and spirits).

Kelly's Directory of Northamptonshire 1885 has an interesting entry. Robinson, William, druggist, stationer, seedsman and various services. These are unspecified except for the extraction of teeth. I wonder if he syringed and pierced ears. This is only the second known reference to dentistry and the last until the 1920 Kelly's Directory (Mrs. George Thompson's property) when Evans, Wm. J. was listed as attending the dental surgery on Fridays.

This long interval does not necessarily mean Long Buckby was poorly served by dentists; only that there are by no means complete sets of Directories.

According to the late Harold Clifton (the former Village historian) Thomas March, H.H. Newitt followed by Edgar Nicholls (married Miss Florence Newitt, daughter of H.H.), A.E. Lemon, K.H. Grace-Dutton (preasent pharmacist) have all occupied the premises still used. These, therefore, have been occupied by a chemist for nearly 150 years (Thomas March; Pigot 1841), or perhaps for rather less if Thomas March Senior practised from somewhere else first.

According to Rate Book, 1841, according to the Form provided and directed to be used by the Poor Law Commissioners (Mr. Fredrick G. Buswell's property). Thomas March Junior (that seems certain) owned his house and shop. Rateable value was £4-4s-0d, at the rate of 15d in the pound his rates were £0-5s-3d.

Mr. Grace-Dutton bought Mr. Lemon's business in 1972.

Details from the Pharmaceutical Register[2] are as follows:- Thomas March registered from 1868-1910 (in business before 1868) – this fits with the 1864 P.O. Directory of Six Counties which lists Mr. March no occupation) and March, Thomas Jnr., druggist and stationer). Died 10th April 1910, Northampton. Herbert Henry Newitt registered from 1874-1901 listed at Long Buckby from 1879. Died 16th December 1901. 1901-1936 – no register of premises.

Details from Register of Premises.

1936 – Representatives of H.H. Newitt

1941 – Edgar Nicholls

1954 – Arthur Edward Lemon.

References:

1. *Concise Oxford Dictionary 5th Edition.* Fell, n, Animal's hide or skin with the hair (also in transferred sense of human skin); thick or matted hair or wool, fleece, (– of hair, unkempt head of hair) -monger. *7th Edition;* Fellmonger – one who prepares skins for leather-making.
2. Letter from The Pharmaceutical Society of Great Britain in reply to one from Mr. K.H. Grace-Dutton.

It seems then, that the Marches established the pharmaceutical tradition in the village, even though T. March Senior had lapsed into hairdressing. No invidious distinction here; after all the early surgeons were solely technicians and allied to the barbers. They had only relatively recently separated from the Company of the Barber-Surgeons.

It can be seen that the Marches were in the mainstream of dispensing. Whether qualified (M.P.S.) or not they were the first to concentrate on pharmacy; they lasted as a business so long, and sold at least one of their own proprietaries. A label for OPODELDOC or SOAP LINIMENT exists describing T. March as Dispensing and Family Chemist, Market Place, Long Buckby.

From the (admittedly) few Commercial Directories examined it seems that the other druggists did not survive long in business and were mainly grocers selling simple medicaments across the counter. John Clark was a fellmonger and may have prepared skins for leather-making by converting raw hide into leather by soaking it in a liquid containing tannic acid; or by use of mineral salts. This would fit with his being a druggist at a time when shoe-making was making headway.

Did John Driver need to make casks to sell drugs in bulk?[1]

It may seem strange at first sight that pharmacy (or at least being a druggist) and stationery were so often associated. I am indebted to Mr. Ken Grace-Dutton for explaining that pharmacy/chemistry was concerned with dyes and inks and naturally led to the sale of stationery. He points out that Boots the Chemists began as a small retail shop in Nottingham undercutting the pharmacists in the sale of simple items such as Epsom Salts and sodii bicarb etc. Jesse Boot was unqualified. His wife worked in the shop which was expanded to employ a qualified pharmacist. Later the business was diversified to sell picture frames, handbags and, inevitably, stationery.

Perhaps the most versatile druggist was Joseph Driver, 1849, whom I turned up in the Trades and Subjects card index at County Records. He was listed as bookseller, stationer, druggist, cooper and pattern maker. He was also in business in West Haddon.[2]

H.H. Newitt bought a Family Grocer's business in 1900 and was advertising in 1902 as a grocer, chemist and stationer.

He had his own lines. Half page advertisements in the Long Buckby Parish Magazine tell us about.

Newitt's Hair Lotion,
1/- per bottle.

Newitt's Cydonia Cream,
6d and 1/- per bottle.

Newitt's Eucalyptus Embrocation,
7½d and 1/1½d per bottle.

As in other spheres the professionals did not always have it all their own way. I am indebted to Mr. Walter Green, sometime Proprietor/Editor of the Daventry Weekly Express, for describing West's Pile Ointment manufactured at 10 Rockhill Road from a secret formula.

All that was known about this popular and efficacious remedy was that Bob and Mary West went for years at the end of the last century, and the beginning of this, to Billing to pick a herb (presumably wild) which was an essential ingredient. The recipe handed down for generations, remained a secret to their deaths.

Of course, seedmen and druggists did not have the monopoly of dental extraction. Blacksmiths would oblige you.

Probably the first reference to dentistry in Long Buckby is in the will of William march, the elder, Weaver, made in 1783 and proved in Northampton on 23rd April 1792. In it, as well as bequeathing his weaving apparatus, he leaves "my Shaving, Bleeding and Tooth-drawing Instruments also my Books and all my Wearing apparel to my son Thomas."

References:

1. John Driver – described in Whellan's Directory 1849, as cooper, drugs and stationery dealer. *Concise Oxford Dictionary*. Cooper, n, (also wine cooper) one who samples, bottles or retails wine; equal mixture of stout and porter; (vt) to stow in casks, to repair (casks). So perhaps he was a wine merchant.
2. Incidentally, J.Castell, at the end of "A Narrative of Some Facts" (concerning the Braunston Cholera outbreak) described himself as Printer, Bookseller, and Druggist, High Street, Daventry. (1835).

6. Within Living Memory

This section must, necessarily, be prosaic compared to some of its predecessors. Gone is the drama; finished are the mighty sanitary battles of late Victorian times. We now enter an era of modern hygiene and sanitation with a District Nurse and Infant Welfare Centre.

Dr. Arthur Cox had died and Dr. W. King Churchouse was taking over from his father. Perhaps the most interesting, possibly unique, feature of this period is that there were two doctors, each the son of a doctor, each following his father in the practice, practising separately. Dr. Ernest Cox and Dr. King Churchouse, both born and bred in the village, were in contemporary, though independent, practice from 1919 (King Churchouse's demobilisation after the First World War) until Ernest Cox's death in 1932.

Ernest Cox not only entered the profession but followed his father to the same Medical School (King's College Hospital, London) and emulated his father in playing his part in local affairs. He was educated at Birkenhead School, played Rugby football for the village, captained the club in his last playing season and was President for 25 years. He was also a cricketer and once distinguished himself in the Long Buckby Tennis Tournament. He found time, too, to act as a School Manager and to be a Director of Long Buckby Gas Co. He was also President of Long Buckby Town Silver Prize Band. He practised from the age of 24 from Holly House, which then had a single story surgery extension projecting at right angles from the High Street front, and died aged 53 after practising about 30 years. By public subscription a bed was endowed in the Manfield Orthopaedic Hospital, Northampton, in his memory.

One local result of the introduction of National Health Insurance in 1913 was that the doctor was obliged to build an extension to the surgery as a waiting room. (Personal communication, the late A.G. Cox, son, and the writer). In exchange for Lloyd George's National Health Insurance Scheme protecting the financial base of general practice by ensuring that at least part of doctors' incomes was guaranteed, facilities for patients were improved.

Again a doctor's son, a northerner from near Barnard Castle in

Teesdale, was to take over. Dr. E.W. Atkinson of Caius College, Cambridge (Hospital not Known) M.R.C.S. (Eng.), L.R.C.P. (London), who had served in the R.A.M.C. during the 'First War' and who had practised at Runcorn, bought the practice though not the house.

First listed in Kelly's Directory of Northamptonshire in 1936, he later moved to a smaller house, 91 High Street, (now 4 East Street), which was to remain the practice premises until well after he retired. He served as M.O. to the Home Guard during the Second World War and died in 1948 or '49.

When released from the R.A.M.C., after the Second World War, Dr. C.V. Oldroyd bought Dr. Atkinson's practice in 1946 or 1947 and continued to use the same house until the joint surgery was completed in the autumn of 1954.

The writer became Assistant with a view to Partnership on October 1st 1948.

To Clifford Oldroyd must go the credit for amalgamating the practices and having the joint surgery built. He was able to convince local councillors that Daventry Rural District Council should be persuaded to build a surgery as an amenity for Long Buckby. It was, therefore, an early example, if not the first in the county, to be specially built by a Local Authority. And it was unusual in having been built by a District Council rather than the County Council.

A perhaps horrifying fact is that there was not a single examination couch in the village for many years. In the old 'Cox' practice from about 1938 (move of premises); in the 'Churchouse' practice from much further back, until the joint surgery was opened in 1954. This was not such a heinous omission as might at first be thought. Cervical smears were not thought of and abdominal and full examinations were carried out at home at arranged visits.

After Franklin Churchouse's death in 1927 the practice was continued from Chard House until the surgery was moved to a wooden building in Southolm garden (King Churchouse's residence) in 1946.

Educated at Oakham School, King Churchouse (Charing Cross Hospital) died aged 61, after 30 years of an almost vanished style of country practice – visiting, branch surgeries and dispensing in the villages.

The hallmark of his practice was personal service, punctuality and availability. He even did a short (slightly later than on weekdays) Sunday morning surgery. And to cater for increased work in the winter he ran a 4.0 - 4.30 pm surgery from 1st October to 31st March. Clifford Oldroyd never held an evening surgery until the joint premises were occupied when both doctors had a 5.30 pm consulting session.

King Churchouse was a fine Regimental Medical Officer, being awarded a Military Cross (M.C.) and three Mentions in Despatches. The last of these was after the end of hostilities and was for public (military) health (Personal communication). This mention worthily upheld his father's tradition of fearless and uncompromising advocacy of preventive medicine.

On King Churchouse's sudden death on the 28th October 1949 the writer was switched, in a day, from assistantship in a non-dispensing practice to being on his own as 'locum' in an entirely strange dispensing practice.

The advent of the National Health Service the previous year had abolished goodwill and sale of practices so the writer was confirmed in the death vacancy of this single-handed practice by Northamptonshire Executive Council, N.H.S., as the doctors' administrative body was then called.

Once again a second generation 'medical' (Newcastle-upon Tyne, Dunelm) had taken over and there was a partnership between two north countrymen.

Clifford Oldroyd retired in 1964.

Dr. N.M How's appointment in June 1964 to the 'Assistantship with a View' and his later attainment of Partnership seems a fitting moment for a younger hand to chronicle more recent events.

7. Personal Recollections

I suppose I am a transitional figure. Transitional because my time in the practice spanned three changes. I began practising during the era of therapeutic barrenness up to the late 1940s and I was to see the exciting explosion of pharmaceutical research and development which produced so many therapeutically effective drugs and antibiotics. I was here when Long Buckby was a relatively small village and was to watch development. Lastly, I began in truly, old-style rural practice and carried over into more modern practice with the accent on clinics and monitoring.

When I was transferred to the other independent practice on the sudden death of King Churchouse I found a very different practice from the one I had been working in for the past year. To begin with it was a dispensing practice, i.e. dispensing for all patients a mile or more from Long Buckby. I had never been a dispensing doctor. It was run on a system of dispensing in the villages, branch surgeries and call houses. Dispensing was fine so long as the Doctor's Winchesters of concentrated stock mixtures lasted out. And I was at first unable to find his formulae! What was not so good was to remember which branch surgery was running low in Mist No. 3 and to remember to take more out.

The reader will appreciate that, while the locum, it was de trop for me to make changes. This was a distinctly single-handed practice without receptionist or dispenser and Mrs. Cynthia Churchouse, who was in hospital at the time of her husband's death, merely took messages and held the 'phone while I was out.

However, as the days shortened I gradually got to know the practice better and became more confident that I was seeing the people who were chronic outlaying patients and who needed me. There was a visiting list but this was complicated by being surnames only in villages which contained several families of the same name.

A period of considerable anxiety and concern was rewarded by being confirmed as principal in the vacancy, and I could make changes. These were inevitably thought of at first as negative although I like to think they were rational.

The first thing I did was to cut out the (later-than-weekdays) Sunday morning surgery. This was not to enable me to attend church but I just felt that, as I worked hard enough all week, I should be allowed a little rest from routine work on Sunday. As it was I was generally working – catching up with correspondence, busying myself checking drug stocks, ordering, making up stock mixtures and, of course, visiting when necessary.

My next, unpopular, change was to close a village surgery about ¼ mile from another one in the twin village of the same parish. Sharing a church and a post office was one thing but sharing a branch surgery was quite another matter; and I was new and had had no introduction. The more branch surgeries there were the more complicated life became and, often, the more difficult it was to keep to time.

Some villages had branch surgeries, some had not. Some only had call houses. I am not sure I didn't prefer the villages with call houses. At least in them one wasn't faced with an unknown number of waiting patients in an already busy winter round. Admittedly one collected several new visits at call houses but one knew the worst at once. Instead there was that first stomach-churning glance into the waiting room and wondering whether there were 8, 10 or a dozen patients and trying to estimate how long the surgery would take.

Of course the call houses had their problems. Depositing medicines, or collecting bottles for refill, was nothing. Call houses were nearly always at chronic patients' homes. So there was a lengthy consultation, or if there wasn't actually one, one was expected to stay a decent time. I was never sure if the selection of a call house resulted from an originally regular, frequent and 'chronic' visit or whether, having chosen the house as a call house the inhabitant became a chronic patient. I never did choose a call house. They were all in place when I came. Branch surgeries were a different matter. I had to alter them; to choose more suitable people or premises.

After appointment, overhaul and modernization of the practice pharmacopoeia had to be undertaken and a better system of distribution of the drugs introduced. I found a reasonable range of tablets for 1949 but the medicines put me in mind of the wartime regimental medical pannier with its tablets numbered from 1 to 10 (No. 9 being widely known as a strong cathartic). In this case it was Mist No. 3, Mist No. 4 and Mist No. 7.

I had no means of knowing whether there had been Misturae Nos. 1 to 7 or more and that a larger number of stock mixtures than I encountered had been whittled down to the therapeutic efficacy of 3; with factors of economy and, possibly, the saving of valuable time and effort being involved. I suspected so.

No. 3 was a stomachic and coloured pink. No. 4 was an all-round cough mixture containing plenty of Tinct Opii Camph; No. 7 was a tonic. I believe there was a Mist Alba, unnumbered and for constipation. There must have been a diarrhoea mixture but it eludes me as it was so long ago. I increased the range. I ceased loading my car with Winchesters, spare bottles, corks and labels and tablets and did all my dispensing centrally. Even when I was taking everything out my car did not quite resemble the boots of modern vets. Many and varied were the agencies and people employed to get medicines out to branches and call houses. These included a village head teacher, a vicar (now the Archdeacon of Oakham), postmen, my wife, myself making a detour next day to drop items at a call house and, latterly, having to make special, out-of-the-way journeys. There must have been other shifts I was put to in order to deliver medicines. This must sound like a chronicle of a bygone age; but in fact it existed until the great British motorised public appeared on the scene and everyone was on the telephone. Certainly without this regular and assiduous village visiting the old and disabled would not have been seen, as rural bus services were inconvenient and friendly, neighbourly cars were not nearly so available.

The best feature that I inherited and which was to stand the test of my time in the practice, was the zoning of the main practice area into visiting rounds. This was conveniently bisected by the A428 (Northampton-Crick) Road which older characters when I first came still called 'The Turnpike'. I used to think of it as the practice main artery and one could branch off it, to left or right, if one wasn't actually doing a round but was going to or from Northampton.

On Monday and Thursday the villages to the south-west of A428 were visited. These were Great and Little Brington, Nobottle if necessary, Upper and Lower Harlestone and return home via A428 often taking in Althorp Park. On Tuesday and Friday East Haddon, Holdenby, The Bramptons and Ravensthorpe – sometimes Spratton – to the north east were visited. I either retraced my steps from Brampton and Holdenby to

Villages covered by practice(s).

go to Ravensthorpe, or, if there were a visit in or near Lower Harlestone, I could come back to Buckby by the A428.

The practice (my part) was not very strong to the north of Long Buckby so there were not many patients in West Haddon and Watford villages. Even so one tried to group these; Buckby calls, Whilton to the south and very outlying families into Wednesday and Saturday.

By this time the reader may well be asking him-or herself how on earth I managed to do it and what about emergencies. All I can say is that there had to be some system – one could not possibly visit every village every day, or even try – because time, effort and finance would have precluded this. Of course there were urgent calls and these naturally took precedence over routine work. Two generations of Churchouses had run the practice this way, the system worked and the patients accepted it. By and large the patients were very helpful and co-operative.

Latterly, when the logistics of medicine delivery became more difficult the Tuesday and Friday routine became modified by dashes to Lower Harlestone (A428 again – I knew every inch of that road) or fast runs across to Great Brington, to deliver medicines before even the proper work of the day had begun.

When Clifford Oldroyd and I amalgamated we still retained our personal lists and ran the two parts of the practice separately even after we had joined forces in the new surgery in 1954. We only saw each other's patients on alternate duty weekends and at nights.

I have said that the main part of my practice was outside Long Buckby on the Northampton side of the village. By rough estimate I had about ¼ and Clifford Oldroyd ¾ of the Buckby patients making me based at one end of the practice. Later on this disparity worried me in view of the fact that I saw fewer patients in our own main village despite offering strictly comparable consulting facilities. It wasn't until I began researching the 19th Century doctors for this account that I found the basis for it. Well before Rural District Councils and more than 75 years before Lloyd George's National Health Insurance (N.H.I.) Scheme, Arthur Cox was appointed Surgeon, Medical Officer and Public Vaccinator to No. 4 District, Daventry Union. This meant he was medically responsible for the poor in No 4 District which included Long Buckby itself, Watford,

Welton Station, Ashby St Ledgers and all this end of the Daventry Union. The boundaries of the old Daventry Union became Daventry Rural District Council and this preponderance of patients perpetuated itself in the N.H.I. of 1913 and in the National Health Service (N.H.S.) of 1948 when everyone could avail themselves of free medical treatment. Similarly Franklin Churchouse (and Fredrick W. Dix before him) was appointed Surgeon, Medical Officer and Public Vaccinator to No. 5 District, Brixworth Union. This included the Bringtons, the Harlestones, the Bramptons, East Haddon, Holdenby and Ravensthorpe, thus eventually giving me more patients in those villages and outside Long Buckby.

Clifford Oldroyd had a virtual monopoly of the village and parish of Ashby St Ledgers and extended over to Welton and Kilsby.

My only achievement during this time, apart from giving dental anaesthetics on Wednesday afternoon at County Hall, Northampton, which added a little spice to life, was to introduce an appointment system for my Long Buckby surgeries. This was about 1960 and we had by then a full morning receptionist who answered the telephone and dispensed as well. She could do the lot which contrasts strongly with to-day's conditions. We also had an evening receptionist but at all other times our wives had to be at home with the practice number switched to the house of the doctor on duty. I was proud to be one of the first doctors to introduce an appointment system. It was a very controversial thing then. "It would never work in my practice". There was much shaking of heads and all I could say when asked about my system and how I justified it was to reply that they should try it and see. Jeffrey Phillips of Daventry (Dr. Clements's partner) just beat me to it but I think I was second in the County to begin one.

It was hard work and I used to get very tired. There wasn't much leisure and in the early years we only took a fortnight's holiday; the weekend roster with the neighbouring practices was in the future. It was a 5½ day week with a normal surgery on Saturday mornings at Buckby plus cold minor surgery under local anaesthesia afterwards if I felt like it and there were cases. The weekend began at 12.00 noon if one wasn't on duty until 9.00 a.m. on Monday. I think what I found so grindingly tiring was the attention to minute detail day after day, month after month, year in year out. It was both mental and physical fatigue, extreme at times, especially at the end of the winter and before the holiday.

So what kept me going? Good question. I hesitate to mention the unfashionable word vocation but, as there were no careers masters at my school, as no one pushed me into medicine; and as it gradually came to me in my 16th year that I should be a doctor, I suppose I had one. But that did not keep me going nor, I am sure, does it keep any general practitioner going. Consultants are different. They have the intellectual stimulus of close contact with colleagues in hospital; they teach and they can keep abreast of new developments in their speciality more easily. For rural practitioners it is different; there is isolation and for me postgraduate education was 10½ miles away in the lunch hour, after evening surgery or sometimes in the afternoons.

Determination and sticking power were certainly necessary. But one also needed inspiration and hope – hope that one could rise to the occasion; hope that one had not declined to a pedestrian level of practice – and this, with inspiration, was provided by the memorable sayings of charismatic teachers at Medical School.

The cause, symptoms and signs, terminations and treatment of inflamation were so drummed into me in hospital before the advent of Penicillin that, when one met it in general practice one fell naturally into the old check-list as though one had never left hospital. Of course treatment changed and became easier with antibiotics but it made one feel good to be so well grounded. And if it came to surgery one wasn't afraid to incise under local anaesthesia – hospital was 10½ miles away. Nevertheless it was good to see the end of serious inflamation and severe skin infections such as boils and carbuncles. The near demise of the staphylococous was a wonderful experience for G.Ps.

I never did hear "the croaking cry of the cretin"[1] but was always hoping to. That honour fell to Nan Thomson (correct spelling *R.G.L.*, Scots) and to her eternal credit she diagnosed it at about 7 weeks. That wonderfully alliterative description was James Spence's of Newcastle[2] and he told us to listen for it every time we opened, or were near, the waiting room door. Not so easy nowadays in modern surgeries when little or no sound emerges from the waiting room. But it was one thing that helped to keep me on my toes.

Let's not be too pretentious about all this. All I am saying is that one must stay sharp. An example of what I mean is well illustrated by the veterinary profession. Some years ago now my children held a party and invited the lady assistant vet at Daventry. As she was walking through our hall she said "that cat has a swollen face". We did not even know the cat was ill. It was curled up relaxed and asleep in an easy chair. Next morning we thought it's face looked a bit swollen. It was developing an abscess.

What does one do when one notices an obvious mysoedema,[3] a colleague's patient, walking along the main street of a village? Should a doctor's mind, or a vet's for that matter, ever be fully switched off? I think not, otherwise he will cease automatically to observe everyone and his alertness will suffer.

This is all very fine when one is not under pressure; but it MUST also apply when one is being swamped by winter work in case the one thing that matters is swamped also by all the colds and 'flu' cases.

Tiredness was an occasion when sharpness could decline. My third call after evening surgery was to a vomiting infant about 7 to 8 weeks old. "What a time to call me out to a feeding difficulty", I thought. "Oh God that baby looks ill and dehydrated, been going on rather a long time", I thought. "And you say the vomit shoots right clear of you"....(to myself), "come on, Lilly, raise your game". ...."Mother, I would like to watch a feed, left breast please". And there it all was – visible peristalsis, the hardening of the pyloric tumour under the pulp of one's left middle finger, followed by the projectile vomit and he passed a green starvation stool into the bargain. A classic pyloric stenosis.[4] In!

Then again there is the slack time; nothing seems to be happening, no problems, and the practice is almost boring. All is going well. This is the time for special alertness or one may be lulled into a sense of false security.

It was a lovely autumn afternoon when I received a call to see a baby "with colic". It was a special visit to a village that I would not ordinarily have visited that day. There was no panic and no seeming urgency. It turned out to be the most memorable clinical afternoon of my life; the day two medical aphorisms were proved true in one day. James Spence had told us in class that we could expect to see one case of acute intussusception of childhood[5] in our professional lives, that it would be atypical and we would miss it. What a challenge! It was Spence's charismatic way of teaching to make us remain aware of it year after year. And I had to wait 25 years for this afternoon. Abdominal examination did not suggest an infant with an acute surgical emergency nor was he in severe distress. "If you don't put your finger in you'll put your foot in it". Stated more formally in lectures that no abdominal examination is complete without a rectal examination. I could feel no tender mass internally; when I withdrew my little finger out came blood in the form of a black currant jelly stool. The diagnosis was made. Without the rectal it would have been missed.

References:

1. Cretin – congenital deficiency of thryroid hormone.
2. Spence, the late Sir James, First Nuffield Professor of Child Health at Newcastle-upon-Tyne.
3. Thyroid deficiency syndrome.
4. Congenital muscular obstruction of the outlet, or pylorus of the stomach.
5. Acute intussusception of childhood – acute telescoping of one length of bowel into another leading to acute intestinal obstruction.

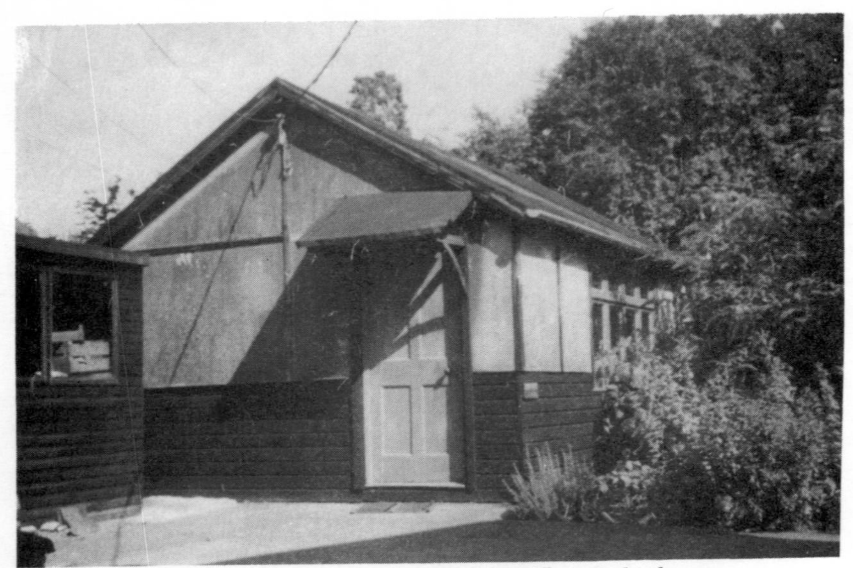

A Rural Surgery – that of Dr. King Churchouse in his later years and that of the author from October 1949 until May 1952

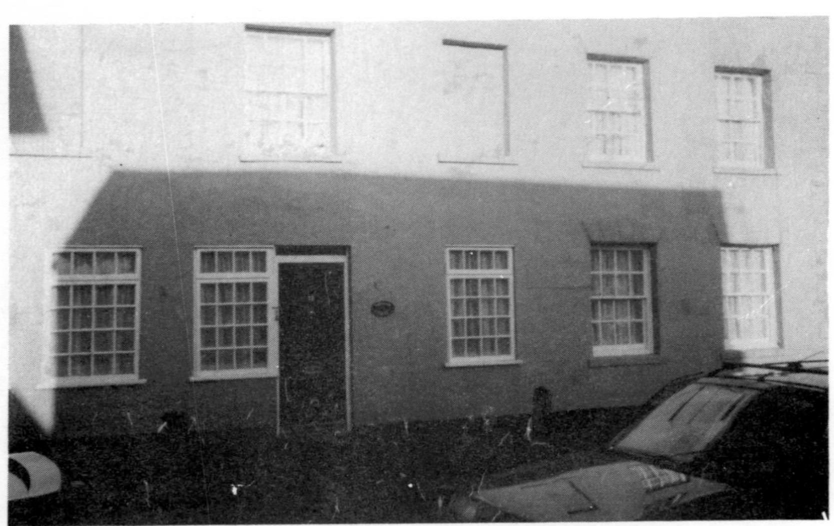

The authors's temporary surgery from May 1952 until the joint surgery opened.

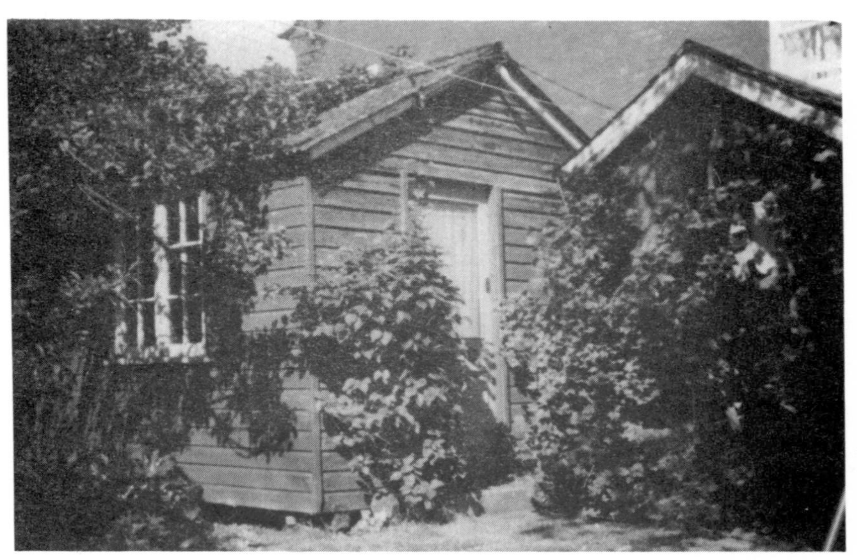

A Rural Surgery – Dr. Atkinson's and Dr. Oldroyd's surgery at 91 High Street (now East Street) Long Buckby, until the joint surgery opened showing doctors' entrance and dispensary.

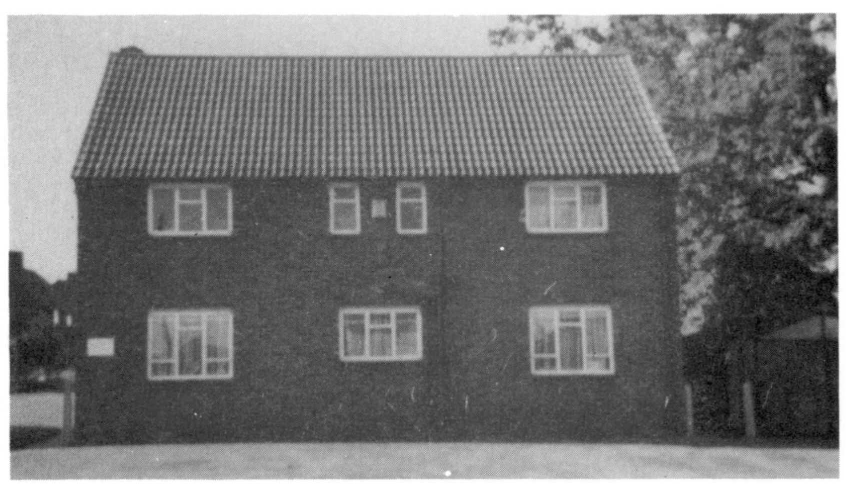

The Joint Surgery opened in October 1954

Appendix I

On page 19 of Waddy's book we read "A Mr. James Gill was appointed Apothecary in 1750. And in June 1753 he was given permission to have an apprentice to be indentured for seven years or at least five years." This takes care of my doubts about Apothecary training in one Voluntary Hospital and I think it is a fair assumption that similar arrangements would have been made in most other 18th Century Charitable Infirmaries.

However, from 1754 onwards Mr. Gill was designated as House Surgeon Apothecary then, later in 1754, when a House Surgeon, an Apothecary, a Secretary and Matron were appointed by the quarterly courts, he remained as House Surgeon and Apothecary. So two separate persons were not appointed.

On page 50 we read the terms for an apprentice.

1st Jan. The Terms proposed are as follows:-

1791 Mr. Foster's Son to be bound to Dr. Kerr for 5 years paying annually in advance £31-10s-0d

To be appropriated as follows:-

To the Hospital for his board	£18-0s-0d
To the Apothecary for the trouble of instructing him	£5-5s-0d
	£23-5s-0d
Remains	£8-5s-0d

By 1804 the fee paid by each apprentice to the House Surgeon Apothecary was still £5-5s-0d.

Langford, in his Presidential Address to the Woolhope (Herefordshire) Naturalists Field Club, stated that, in the original rules of the Hereford General Infirmary (founded 1776), each physician was allowed:

> "To take two pupils, and only two at one time, being members of an University (my underlining) and to receive a satisfactory gratuity from them for their instruction in attending the infirmary; but that no such pupil shall be permited to prescribe in any case."

The same rule applied to the Surgeons, with the variation that:

> "No pupil or apprentice shall perform any operation, but shall have liberty to dress a patient under the direction of his master."

It seems perfectly plain to me that the physicians' pupils were post-graduates with medical theory attending Hereford General Infirmary for clinical experience.

In support of this, and more specifically, we read in a book of Northampton Infirmary Sermons 1744-1748, beautifully bound in red morocco and kindly loaned to me by the late Victor Hatley, Rule 7. of the Rules concerning the Physicians. "That the Physicians in Ordinary be permitted the Liberty (usual in most Hospitals) of taking Pupils to be instructed in Physick, and of receiving from them a satisfactory Gratuity, provided such Pupils are, or have been, Members of the Universities of Oxford or Cambridge: And that these pupils attend the patients of that Physician only to whose Instruction they have committed themselves (unless otherwise agreed on by the Physicians;) but that the Pupil be on no Occasion suffered to prescibe."

There is still one slight mystery left. What is the difference between a Surgeon's Pupils and his apprentice? Rule 7. of the Rules concerning the Surgeons reads "That each Surgeon be allowed to have only two Pupils, and one Apprentice, to attend the Hospital, and that they be permitted to take money for the informing of such Pupils, or Apprentice: But that no Pupil or Apprentice attempt under Pain of immediate expulsion, to perform any operation, except Bleeding, making a Seaton *(Oxford Concise* Seton), or cutting an Issue, and even that by Order of one of the Surgeons; and that they do not presume to dress, or take off any Dressing, unless one of the stated Surgeons be present." So they were very closely supervised.

The difference in status was probably one of seniority and length of training; the pupils having completed their apprenticeships and being in the nature of journeymen – qualified but not yet fully experienced and still working for another – though paying for the privilege. The apprentice was younger and had begun his training at fifteen under the surgeon.

The Surgeons were forbidden to dispense or administer medicine.

Rule 11. of The Physicians' Rules reads "....but that no Internal Medicines shall be administered by the Surgeons or be dispensed by the Apothecary, but with the Direction of a Physician; unless on Casualties when Patients are suddenly brought in or where a Chirurgical Case instantly requires the Administration of Internal Medicines, at a time when the Physicians cannot be conveniently consulted."

Appendix II

Since my account went into typescript, attention has been drawn by the late Victor Hatley to the following announcement reproduced in photocopy and printed below. It appeared in the *Northampton Mercury* dated 29th October 1791.

HORSE-MARKET, NORTHAMPTON.

THE flattering Encouragement I have met with in my Profeſſion, (eſpecially in this Neighbourhood,) during the five Years I have had the Honour to practice in it, hath led me to believe that a Reſidence in the reſpectable Town of Northampton would be highly eligible for my future Expectations, (my Leaſe at Long-Buckby expiring Lady-Day next,) for which Purpoſe I have purchaſed the Houſe lately occupied by Mr. Lockwood, in the Horſe-Market, and have this Day opened the ſame; where thoſe who pleaſe to honour me with their Commands, either in MEDICINE or MIDWIFERY, may be aſſured that the greateſt poſſible Attention will be paid to every Caſe committed to my Care.

Great at all Times hath been my Deſire to attain that Degree of Knowledge in my Profeſſion, as to be TRULY uſeful to thoſe who place Confidence in me; for which great End, much Pains have been taken, and very conſiderable Expences incurred by me: over and above that of having regularly attended *the Lectures of the Profeſſors* GREGORY *and* CULLEN, on the *Theory* and *Practice* of *Phyſic*, MONRO and BLACK, on *Anatomy* and *Chemiſtry*, in the *juſtly celebrated Univerſity of Edinburgh*, which at preſent is the *firſt School* for teaching Medicine, &c. in the known World; have alſo received all neceſſary Inſtructions in MIDWIFERY from the firſt Gentlemen in that Profeſſion in London, viz. *Drs.* ORME *and* LOWDER,—attended the Whole of their public *Lectures*,—all the *Labours* that happened (during two Months) in their extenſive *Lying-in Hoſpital*,—*delivered ſeveral Women* (by their Appointment) at private Houſes,—with a Certificate of the ſame given under their Hands and Seals.

Thus qualified, I hope for a Continuance of that Degree of public Confidence, Countenance, and Support, I have hitherto been indulged with. How far I have merited public Favour, by affording Benefit to the Afflicted, is not for me to ſay, but will be beſt known from Patients themſelves. Have only to add, that by an unremitted Attention to the Duties of my Profeſſion, I hope to meet the entire Approbation of my Employers.

October 29th, 1791. J. BLISSARD.

I found no mention of Blissard in the many Long Buckby medical references. The announcement gives a good idea of the advertising prevalent, and presumably common, at the end of the 18th century.

The General Medical Council (G.M.C.) was far into the future.

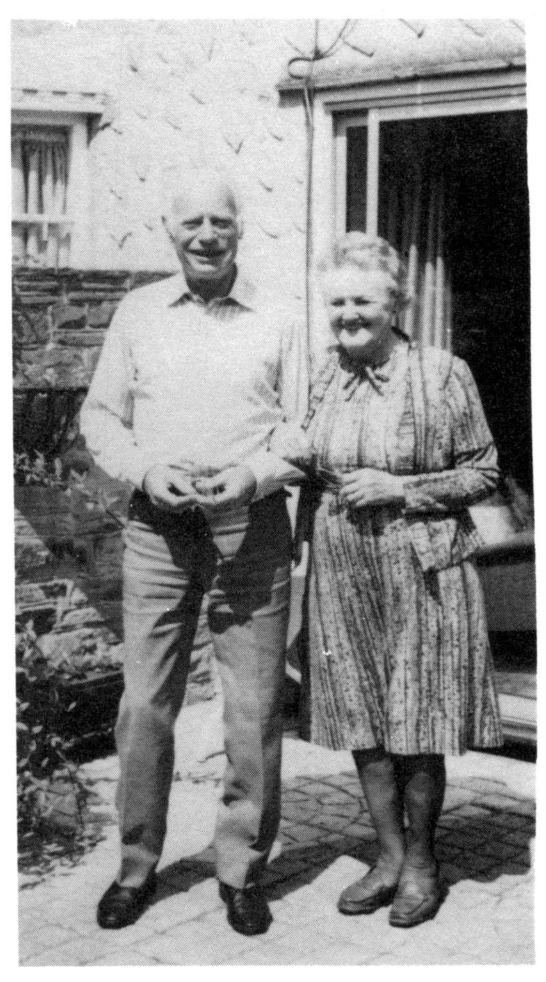

Dr. Graham Lilly with his wife Marie

Polly and Alice

by Winifred Mary Ruston

This book mentioned by the author in his introduction, is about Long Buckby, Crick and Barby.

Originally conceived as a children's story about life in and around these villages and published as Part I. There was obviously a very interesting background and this became Part II.

The picture of village life is at a time of change from an agricultural to an idustrial society and is illustrated with drawings and photographs – the earliest being 1816.

To the reader who wishes to learn more about the times covered by Dr. Lilly's researches, this book provides a rare insight into a community centred on Long Buckby which, unusually for villages in the latter part of the twentieth century, is still a bustling village with shops, a school, etc.

The first edition was published in 1990 and subsequently sold out which led to a second and enlarged edition in 1992.

ISBN 1 870127 65 X (160 pp) Price £3.95

Helpi your child through separation and divorce

CW00597139

Published by Collins Dove
A Division of HarperCollins*Publishers* (Australia) Pty Ltd
22–24 Joseph Street
Blackburn, Victoria 3130

© Copyright Glenda Banks 1981, 1994
All rights reserved. Except where allowed under Australian copyright law, no part of this book may be reproduced without permission in writing from the publishers.

First published 1981
Reprinted 1981, 1988, 1990
Second edition 1994

Designed by Pier Vido
Cover design by Pier Vido

Typeset by Collins Dove

National Library of Australia
Cataloguing-in-Publication data:

Banks, Glenda
Helping your child through separation and divorce.

2nd ed.
ISBN 1 86371 263 1.

1. Children of divorced parents. I. Title.

306.89

1

What to expect when your partner walks out

'If only I'd known what to expect, I might have handled things better . . . '

Psychiatrists and psychologists hear this phrase repeated more than any other by the emotional casualties of separation and divorce. It is the excuse most frequently offered by parents in relation to the emotional abuse suffered by their children.

Here, we take the normal progression of the trauma step-by-step, so that you will be prepared for your own reactions and can reserve enough of your emotional resources through the harrowing time ahead to help your child through separation and divorce.

Many survivors of the separation and divorce trauma agree that unless a marriage is terminated amicably, with prior agreement reached over custody and access and the division of property and assets, there are four phases through which one or both partners must pass before the trauma subsides and each can carry on to live independently of the other. These are: the denial phase, the critical phase, the identity crisis, and the mourning phase.

The main thing to keep in mind as you progress through each one is that it will not last for ever. It may not be replaced by relief—indeed, the next phase, by comparison with your life prior to separation may seem a lot worse, but that will pass, too. And, at the end of the separation and divorce trauma, you may well find you have developed a whole new approach to life . . . a formula for living *on your own terms* instead of merely existing in someone else's shadow.

No one can pretend the months ahead are going to be easy, or that you can approach them with confidence, even if you are forewarned. There will probably be times when you feel you cannot carry on for another hour, let alone another day, or month, or year. You may also become so bitterly disillusioned by the attitudes of those around you (your former partner in particular) that you feel you might as well give up and give in to whatever demands are made upon you. And there will be periods when your own behaviour makes you seriously begin to question your own sanity.

But you can survive. If you take one phase at a time, examine it, sort it out into sections and tackle them one by one, as if you were working on a project to be dealt with as part of a course in human survival—and what else is it, when all is said and done?—you can gradually see it through to the end with a sense of purpose and self worth which provides the strength you need to achieve your goal: the emotional survival of yourself and your child.

The denial phase

Separation is the worst period of the whole divorce trauma. Everything is new and raw, and your own reactions are entirely self destructive. So much has changed so quickly that you are left with few familiar points of reference. Your timing is out, with no partner around whom to gear your day, and no high points of stimulation to look forward to—even if you did argue when he (you) came home from work.

Even though your partner has set up a home for himself

elsewhere, you refuse to accept the fact that the marriage is over, however bad your relationship and whoever he may have lined up to replace you. You lie awake at night and drift through your day trying to work out where the marriage fell apart, and how to put it back together again. You look for answers in changes you might make to the peripheral aspects of the marriage: perhaps you could get back together again if your husband changed his job, or you gave up yours . . . if you could win the lottery and write off your money worries . . . if your child went to kinder, and you weren't so tired all the time.

But you are wasting your time. Rarely does a change of circumstance bring a couple together permanently, so soon after the break-up. If you are not careful, this is the time you can get caught in a no-man's land of conjecture, of maudlin dreams about the past and what might have been in the future. Human nature can play tricks; we have a tendency to remember only the good things about the past. Thus, in most cases, conjecture about proposed changes in circumstances surrounding your marriage must fail if put to the test. For you will have left the basic weaknesses of your marriage out of your formula for success, and with the added stress of change, it is sure to break down again.

The denial phase can last months, even years. Indeed, some women refuse to accept a marriage is over long after their husbands have married new partners, and continue to live a quasi-married existence for the rest of their lives. Some do this for their children in the belief that, if the second marriage fails and the husband returns to his original family, the disruption will have been minimal. Others cling for religious reasons.

If you are considering this, coasting or waiting it out to see if your husband has a change of heart, forget it. Even if you do get together again, you cannot pick up the threads of the old marriage and carry on as if nothing has changed, and neither can your child. The split would never have occurred if the old marriage had been tolerable.

Ergo, it has to change. And so do you. No one can go through the trauma of separation without changing, and those changes must affect the tenor of the marriage if you decide to continue it.

Usually, the decision to accept the break-up as final is made for you. Your husband takes a job in another city, state or overseas, or moves in with a new partner, or you have to leave your family home so that it can be sold to effect the property settlement and you know, whatever you do, it won't be enough to put it all together again. End of phase one . . .

The critical phase

Now you are on your own. This is the end of hoping, planning, dreaming, trying for two, and you are at rock bottom, emotionally.

Your predominant reactions at this time will be depression, anger and guilt. The depression may well manifest itself as physical illness or, at least, extreme fatigue. Being pushed to one's limits emotionally can be just as depleting as being pushed to the limits physically. But, for some reason, we tend to ignore or refuse to accept the symptoms of fatigue when they are brought on by emotional exertion; it is as if we have to justify tiredness with something tangible, like a five-mile walk, or we feel we are failing, falling short of some undefined social standard. But you don't have to justify your fatigue or ill health as a result of the toll the crisis is taking of you emotionally. Fatigue is a symptom of your condition just as much as a pain or a persistent cough. Take notice of your body's warning signal and ask your family doctor for his advice.

Sound sleep, the best antidote to fatigue, is probably eluding you at nights, now, just when you need it most. Before you reach for the sedatives and tranquillisers (which, when used properly, and with caution, provide a bridge across the trauma until one can deal with a personal crisis but all too often become a habitual prop which can leave you limping for ever) try a few old fashioned remedies for insomnia. Honey in hot milk, a soothing warm bath, a late, late movie on television, a couple of chapters of some escapist novel, or yoga or deep-breathing exercises—anything to take your mind off your problems and leave it in neutral for a while, as a prelude to sleep.

If insomnia or any other symptom of depression, anxiety or general ill health persists, do see your doctor. It is vital to your ability to cope, for yourself and your child, that you stay in the best possible health for the critical time ahead. It is a good idea to review your eating habits, now, too, for the same reason. You may not feel like eating much but make what you *do* eat count.

Breaking through the depression and fatigue now may be anger—the deep, vengeful 'why did you do this to me (and our child)' type of anger. Your former partner may also experience anger at this time but he will probably interpret the blame as yours, with the 'why did you make me do this to you (and our child)' rationale. That is why physical violence may be a very real risk at this stage, whenever the two of you meet to discuss a divorce or hand over your child for access visits. As a preventative measure, you may find it wise to arrange for a third adult to be present in the house, if not the room, whenever your former partner visits.

You will both be experiencing strong feelings of guilt about now, too. 'Perhaps if I'd done this or that, things might not have gone so wrong . . . ' or 'what am I (are we) doing to our child . . . ?' are common expressions of guilt during the critical phase of separation and divorce.

Guilt is often the motivating factor behind the many desperate attempts at reconciliation which are made during the critical phase, and you may expect many and repeated long, late night phone calls, late night visits and vigils, and many temporary reconciliations, with extremely emotional sexual activity. Couples come together, make love, fight, walk out, come back, make love, move out and so on. In most cases, this is due to the combined effects of guilt and the desperate need to justify what you have done or intend doing to end the marriage. A sort of 'I don't want this to happen but you can see it's hopeless' statement, acted out for the benefit of both partners as a self inflicted wound.

In some cases, the peak activity of the critical phase is a last, genuine effort to make the marriage work, to try to find some spark which might ignite old fires and put warmth back into a cold relationship, or simply to find some level plane on which the marriage might rest until it can be repaired.

Sadly, due to the emotional state of both partners during this period, the prospects for a successful, lasting reconciliation are not good, however well intentioned both partners might be. But this is not to say attempts to reconcile your differences and find some fragment on which, with help, you may be able to rebuild your relationship, should not be made. There is, always, the *chance* a reconciliation could work . . . and there are probably hundreds of thousands of married couples who could tell of brink-of-divorce reconciliations which put their marriage breakdown into perspective as a 'bad patch' which they overcame and built on to work out a better plan for peaceful coexistence, which eventually brought rich rewards.

But don't expect too much of yourself, or your partner, at this stage. See these reconciliation attempts for what they usually are—conscience cleansing exercises which have to be performed if you are not to be cramped by doubt later on.

The identity crisis

With the last hopes of reconciliation extinguished, you face an identity crisis. This occurs as a result of two signals your mind is putting out at the same time: one consciously, the other subconsciously. On the outside, the absence of your partner forces you to face the fact that you are operating now as a single entity, while inside, you still feel the same as you did when your partner was with you. The conflict plays havoc with your emotional and practical reactions to everyday situations, from paying the electricity bill to what to buy to eat, from what to wash first to what time to go to bed. Although you may think you make an instant decision, there is a micro-second's hesitation left over from all the years of considering your partner's needs, desires and preferences.

While individual reactions to this 'dual personality' vary, there is evidence to suggest a general desire to shrug off all ties with a former partner once the break-up has been accepted. Often, this is attempted by surface changes which are quite out of character, affecting your attitudes and behaviour until you become the antithesis of the person you once were, in so far as that reminds you of your relationship with your former husband.

Whatever he liked, you'll want to change, from the way you do your hair to what you watch on TV; from the toilet soap you use to what, and when, you eat. If your marriage lasted some years, it is likely you will try to retrace those years and find out what you missed by being married, either to prepare yourself to get back into the 'race' or to compensate yourself for all the (now) wasted years when you willingly missed so much.

You may find yourself acting out roles, modelled on stereotypes you see around you or on television, trying them on, tossing them off, with a bewildering lack of concern for public opinion or personal consequences. If you stop to consider it, it's almost like going through adolescence all over again; trying to discover who you really are, after all this time being half of someone else. And, like adolescence, your new identity crisis will be peaked with emotional highs and troughed with lows; your mood will swing from elation to despair, with exhausting periods of self analysis in between.

You may also find that this is the time when—much as you love and want him with you—you resent your child. This is not, as one might suppose, because he reminds you of your former partner, or is a common bond you wish to cut loose, but because the demands he makes on your time are a constant reminder of what you really are—a parent, with all the responsibilities that role entails—as well as whoever you wish to be.

One of the most common reactions of men and women caught in the identity crisis is to alter their appearance, quite drastically. Women may change the colour of their hair, will almost certainly change the style, experiment with radically different make-up, clothes and accessories, and sometimes even adopt a whole new moral outlook.

Men most often alter their clothes, affecting a more youthful, modern image, with accentuated fashion trends and out of character accessories, such as a two-door coupe in place of the family wagon or suburban four-door sedan.

Both men and women tend to react against their established choice of partner when it comes to choosing new ones (which are usually temporary at this time). If your husband is tall, dark and handsome, you will probably go for new partners who are short, blond and 'interesting' . . . if your husband likes spectator sports, you will probably look for a man who prefers to spend his Saturday afternoons at an art gallery.

Perhaps the most difficult personality change you may experience during the identity crisis is a new (albeit temporary) moral outlook. If you were a devoted, faithful wife with a highly developed sense of moral values, you may suddenly find you are not only willing but *wanting* to go to bed with the first, half-way tolerable man who asks you. On the other hand, if you 'played up' now and then during marriage, you may find physical advances abhorrent and reject them completely. Men and women report their first experiences of personal impotence or frigidity during the post break-up identity crisis, usually caused by strong feelings of latent fidelity!

A common side effect of the identity crisis, with its peculiar personal behaviour and generally unsuccessful physical encounters (which even if physically stimulating are seldom emotionally satisfying), is the almost overwhelming desire to pay back or get even with your former partner for putting you in this position by shattering your self confidence and causing you to question everything about yourself.

This is the time when you may seriously doubt your own sanity. You may consider schemes which are totally out of character, so at odds with your normal behaviour that you think you are losing your mind. There seems to be no plan too petty, too weird, too savage as you plot the ultimate destruction of the person you may once have protected with your own life.

Among the most common forms of payback or revenge is harassment by telephone, particularly at your former partner's place of employment, or late at night, when he may be sleeping or, possibly, making love with someone else. Even if you have never uttered a single obscenity before, you may find yourself screaming a whole string of obscenities into the mouthpiece of your telephone, over and over again. (You may also be the victim of this form of payback abuse.)

Normally sane and rational women have done worse things to their former partners. One cut the seams of all her former partner's suits the morning before he came to collect them from the family home . . . another took a screwdriver and scratched 'bastard' on the boot of her estranged husband's new car . . . and yet another gave away all his personal possessions, from his pyjamas to his expensive power tools, before her former partner had a chance to arrange for their collection.

Husbands who have quit the family home get hooked on payback, too, even though the decision to quit may have been their own. One husband, disenchanted with his new found bachelor 'freedom', made a point of hammering on his former wife's door when she moved into a new flat of her own, in an effort to disrupt her social life . . . another hired a bulldozer and driver to smash down the family home he'd left, while his wife was out.

The identity crisis phase, with its payback side effect, can last from about eight to twelve months, depending on your resilience and your basic self confidence. And, because you are likely to behave completely out of character, this period is probably the worst for your child, as he will have difficulty relating to someone he often cannot recognise.

To add to his feelings of insecurity, he is probably being shuttled back and forth between you and his other parent, who may be equally unfamiliar and unrecognisable in his own identity crisis. Already extremely unsettled by the departure of one parent from the family home, your child may be in desperate need of reassurance that you will not leave him, too. Sadly, because you and his other parent are stretched to your emotional limits right now, trying to cope with your own reactions, you may not have enough of an emotional reserve left to answer your child's request for emotional support.

The only way your child can communicate his insecurity is through his behaviour. He may be irritable, or whine, or demand you play with him, or simply hang around, clutching at your skirts, generally getting in your way. Or he may argue, challenge you on a variety of ordinary, everyday issues, from what he has to eat for breakfast to what time he has to go to bed, from what he wears to whether or not he cleans his teeth after dinner. Some children develop finely timed temper tantrums which they trot out just before you take them out, or leave them with a baby-sitter or at their creche, kinder or school.

Because this sort of behaviour is new to you, or you are so immersed in your own problems, you may not be able to regard it objectively and look for the *real* cause behind the obvious triggers for your child's emotional outbursts. Not surprisingly, just at the time when you and your child most need love and comfort from each other, you may find you are poles apart. Child abuse, in the physical sense, is a very real danger during this period.

As if all this emotional conflict, within and around you, were not enough, you will also have to contend with the cumulative pressures of the technicalities and legalities of your impending divorce throughout this phase. You may also find yourself in severe financial difficulties as a result of the withdrawal of the main source of income for yourself and your child, so you are probably trying to find part or full-time employment.

But things do gradually resolve themselves, and the divorce itself comes, as a rule, as something of a relief, an anti-climax, according to those single parents who have survived the transition. You then enter the fourth, and final phase of the separation and divorce trauma . . .

The mourning phase

Whether you still love your former partner or have learned, by now, to loathe him, divorce is still the death of your relationship and all the hopes of happiness that went with it. And along with any relief you may feel that the whole horrible business of killing it is done with, you will almost certainly find yourself mourning your loss.

The schism is sudden, even though you have been preparing for it for so long. You feel your new 'separateness' as keenly as an amputation of one of your own limbs, or the sudden death of someone you assumed would always be there. But there are soothing rituals which follow the death of a loved one and help to ease the loneliness. Not the least of these is sympathy from those around you. There is also the time-honoured tradition of funeral arrangements, including a 'wake' or gathering of friends who expect you to blurt out all your fears and anxieties as well as talk of your loss.

After divorce, there is nothing . . . As yet, there are no time-honoured traditions to see you through; no set pattern to follow in the long nights ahead. In place of sympathy, you will more often encounter embarrassment. Instead of being willing to listen to your fears and anxieties, your friends will probably be bored or uncomfortable if they bother to listen at all.

But you are entitled to grieve, nonetheless, for you have lost something, even if it was only an illusion. So go ahead and cry, feel sorry for yourself. Dig up any good memories you might be able to salvage from your dream and savour them. And gradually, as you do after mourning the loss of one who dies a clinical death, you will come out of this final phase all the better for having grieved and got it out of your system.

Some people have described the post divorce period as similar to convalescence after a long illness. The first time you get up out of bed, the floor seems a long way down, your legs are shaking and there is always the chance you will stumble and fall, or have a relapse. But there is no denying, as time goes on, you do feel better. And with a little help, the chances are good that you will eventually make a complete recovery, give or take the odd, fleeting memory. Equally important, so will your child . . .

2

What to tell your child—and how

The walk out, either by one parent alone, or by one parent with the child(ren) of the marriage, seldom occurs without warning. The symptoms of a marriage breakdown—rows, tears, recriminations and possibly physical violence—have probably been witnessed by your child for some months, perhaps years. And yet, there is a natural tendency to shut him out of the family crisis at its peak; to ignore him when he most needs explanations and reassurance.

Psychiatrists and paediatricians agree that to a child, fear of the unknown is often more terrifying than even the most catastrophic actuality, especially if he feels that the family, which is his basic security, is threatened.

There are many case histories on record of the long term effects of keeping a child 'in the dark' about his parents' divorce. Some children build up fantasies to carry them through their own part of the separation–divorce trauma . . . others turn on one or both parents after apportioning blame based on a child's-eye view of events without benefit of adult interpretation . . . even more tragically, some children blame themselves for the breakdown of their parents' marriage and walk out themselves, carrying their 'guilty' secret with them for the rest of their lives.

But how does one tell a child about the breakdown of a marriage? How far should you go back? How can a child possibly comprehend the complexities of the gradual disintegration of the emotional and physical relationship between a husband and wife?

There seem to be two predominant schools of thought on the 'how to tell a child' issue. The first, which is based on the cow-pen philosophy of telling it *all*, with no holds barred because 'a child's got to learn about life sooner or later', has a growing number of supporters as it dispels the need for subterfuge and half truths which can add to a child's confusion if he suspects he is being 'conned'.

But the flaw in that theory is obvious: rarely, if ever, will two warring parents tell the same version of the truth. Each will have his/her own interpretation of the shaping up of the breakdown, the contributing factors, the *real* cause of the current crisis. So the child in the middle will probably receive conflicting stories from the two people he trusts most in the world, and, to add to his bewilderment, he will find his loyalty put to the test when he is forced to accept one version or the other.

The alternative, and equally prevalent attitude is to tell a child the truth—to a point. A prime example of the truth-to-a-point philosophy is the 'daddy's gone away' concept. There are several variants of this, the most popular being: 'daddy's taken a job a long way away and we have to stay here' or 'daddy loves someone else more than he loves us and has gone to live with her' or 'daddy is dead'. (These variants are employed with 'mummy' substituted for 'daddy' when the custodian parent is the father . . .)

The flaws in this philosophy hardly need to be spelled out, either. Unless you tell your child why his daddy really went away, there is every chance he will assume the blame himself—it must have been something he did, felt or wished, that caused daddy to go. If you show anger or grief at the mention of daddy's name thereafter, your child may assume responsibility for that, too, so you have compounded the original problem—coming to terms with the loss of his father.

The short and long term effects of the 'daddy is dead' story can be quite devastating. The shock generated by the death of someone near and dear to a child is often underestimated by adults, especially when a child is first introduced to death. The finality of the end of life (in physical terms) may not be grasped fully until he reaches, say, 10 or 11 years, but the grief occasioned by his sense of personal loss can be overwhelming. Further, your 'grief' (which is how your child may read your tears of anger, humiliation, frustration, fatigue or fear of the future) will probably inhibit him from allowing his grief to show, for fear of making you even more upset. So you've answered none of his questions with the 'daddy is dead' routine, and added the burden of unnecessary grief to his load.

As for the long term effects, curiosity often gets the better of a 'dead' daddy when his child graduates from college or university, reaches 21 or marries. His 'reincarnation' at any of these critical stages in an emerging adult's life can cause your child to seriously question his own *raison d'être*, as well as his father's. And you could pay for your own part in the deception by forfeiting the love and trust you have carefully nurtured in your child over the years since your divorce.

This is not to say that the tell-it-all and the truth-to-a-point theories are entirely without merit. There are elements of sensitivity and sound common sense in each approach to telling your child about the breakdown of your marriage. The trick is to sort through them both for a formula which satisfies your child's need to know what is going on, but doesn't overload him with more than he can digest.

There is a charming story which, although it has been around for some time, serves well to illustrate the overload trap as applied to the modern divorce phenomenon.

Scenario: Six-year-old boy comes into the kitchen where his mother is shelling peas. 'Mother', says the little boy, 'Where do I come from?' His mother, prepared since the moment of his conception, by tomes of advice about how to impart the secret of life to a wondering infant when the magic moment arrives, pauses only long enough to put down her pea pod before launching into the whole routine, from the momentous meeting of sperm and ovum, through all the embryonic stages, right up to the miracle of birth. 'There, darling', she breathes. 'Does that answer your question?' 'Mmmm', replies her son doubtfully, 'Billy says he comes from Melbourne . . . '

A general rule might be: don't bite off more than your child can swallow.

How much you tell your child about the cause and effect of the separation and divorce must depend, to a great extent, on his age and his capacity for understanding. Whatever his age, you should avoid the temptation to tell him everything in one hit. This may unburden and absolve you, but you run the risk of overloading your child to the point at which he switches off completely, and either doesn't hear you or rejects whatever you try to tell him about those issues which are of most interest to him—his continued relationship with his father (mother), your new relationship with his father (mother), and the future as it affects you all.

More importantly, perhaps, if you do tell him too much, too soon, he may reject you for inflicting all this pain upon him—and then he will have no one close, to whom he can turn for the comfort and direction he badly needs right now.

A child's natural loyalty to both parents must also be taken into consideration when you break the news that one or other of you is moving out of the family home. However justified you may feel you are in revealing the true character of your former partner (at least, as you see it), care should be taken not to put your child in the position of having to make judgements. Character assassinations can only leave him feeling doubly bereft; not only has his father (mother) left him, but he cannot even cherish his (her) memory.

Family therapists evaluating the effects of children's reactions to the separation and subsequent divorce of their parents also warn that the *way* a parent, or parents, break the news to their child is as important as the words they use to do it.

All too often when dealing with children, adults give out two conflicting signals. One is transmitted verbally, the other comes across as a body signal. The simplest illustration of dual signalling in common usage is when a parent----mother or father—is obviously upset, either tearful or irritable, and a child asks what is wrong. 'Nothing', the parent replies, leaving the child utterly confused, for what the parent *says* is in direct contrast to what the child *sees* via the body signal the parent is sending out.

Thus, there is little point in pouring out verbal platitudes if your body is signalling the end of the world. If you can't help crying when you explain about the break-up, tell your child you are upset, let him see it's okay for him to be upset too, and he will be able to accept what is happening far more easily because he knows instinctively that you are playing it straight with him.

Whatever and however you decide to break the news about the marriage breakdown to your child, it is vital to his peace of mind and healthy emotional development that you tell him *something* as soon as the split occurs. The following two case histories show what can happen if you leave your child in limbo too long . . .

Jamie was a bright, nine-year-old boy with above average intelligence, who attacked his class work with enthusiasm, was popular with his peers and liked by his teachers. But over a period of three or four weeks, his teachers noticed a surprising change in Jamie's behaviour. Instead of enthusiasm, he exhibited lethargy; instead of attacking his class work intelligently, he affected indifference to the challenge and his marks. And in the playground, the formerly friendly boy became a loud mouthed bully, threatening anyone who earned his disfavour with a walloping from his father.

He also came late to school each day, spoiling a near perfect record for time and attendance. Each day he arrived after the assembly bell, he delivered a new excuse involving his father: his father's car wouldn't start . . . his father couldn't find his office papers . . . his father had slept in.

One morning, Jamie's grade teacher herself arrived late, just in time to see Jamie dawdling along the street outside the school, on foot, with no sign of his father. During the lunch break, the teacher telephoned Jamie's mother to try to find out why he was late and what might be responsible for his change of attitude.

It was then that she learned that Jamie's father had left the family home a month before, after discovering his wife's casual affair with a co-worker. The mother, hoping she could persuade her husband to return, had delayed telling Jamie about the break-up, allowing him to believe that daddy was away on a trip.

As the days went by with no word from his father, or any sign of his return, Jamie invented a scheme to cover his hurt and sense of loss: he created the illusion that his father was still part of the family, still there to share Jamie's life. Hence the excuses involving his father when he was late, and the threats to the other children, supported by his fantasy father. But the strain of keeping the fantasy alive took its toll of the nine year old . . . emotionally and physically. And this accounted for his lack of enthusiasm and attack in his class work.

As soon as Jamie's parents realised what they had inadvertently done to their son, they put aside their differences and became, once more, loving and supportive parents. But Jamie's insecurity went so deep that it took months of careful, professional counselling to coax him back into a 'normal' behaviour pattern.

At the other end of this age scale, the parents of a thirteen year old girl delayed announcing their separation to their daughter, hoping she would get used to the idea of daddy living away from home before the blow fell. They encouraged this by allowing her to believe he was interstate on business for a few months.

In reality, the father had moved only across town, and in view of the amicable atmosphere in which the separation and anticipated divorce was to be conducted, he hadn't bothered to move his bank account to a branch in his new locale.

Inevitably, Sue spotted her father's car outside the family bank one morning during her mid-term break. Delighted at his apparent surprise return home, she waited beside the car to surprise her father in turn. But, sadly, the surprise was all Sue's as her father emerged from the bank with his arm around a young woman holding a new baby in her arms . . .

Such was the girl's humiliation and sense of betrayal, on behalf of her mother as much as herself, at being replaced in the father's affections by the young woman and her baby (Sue's interpretation of events, but with no explanations forthcoming from her parents a perfectly natural assumption for a girl her age), that she ran away rather than face her mother with the news.

The youth worker assigned to help her through her crisis, told how she had been found, some days later, living in the back of a panel van, owned by a youth she had met in an amusement arcade where she had gone to keep warm the night she ran away . . .

Ideally, both parents should try to get together long

enough to work out what, how and when to tell their child about their separation and their plans for his future. Some counsellors believe parents should present the explanation jointly. Others feel the risk of open confrontation between them is too great at the time their child most needs to be reassured of their joint interest in him and his future.

Ideals, however, are rarely attained. And given the emotional state of most parents at the point of separation it is probably more realistic to suggest that you aim to agree on the basic story and when to tell it, then tell it separately, each attempting to reinforce the other's assurances of continued love and concern for the welfare of your child.

Of course, one cannot overlook the possibility that the relationship between a separating couple can deteriorate to such a degree that there is simply no way they can communicate on anything—even the immediate emotional welfare of their child. If this is the situation in which you find yourself, or your former partner opts out of the responsibility altogether (for the time being, anyway), you can either solicit the support of an intermediary or make the decision to go it alone.

It is undoubtedly in your child's best interests to inform his other parent of your intentions regarding the delivery of the explanation your child deserves, if only to give him the opportunity to co-operate later on. You may be able to get the gist of your story across through a third person—a mutual friend or relative whom you both trust.

If you make the decision to do it alone, you can provide valuable back-up support for yourself and your child by inviting a grandparent or some other close relative your child loves and trusts to sit in on the announcement. In the absence of his other parent, your child can draw strength and reassurance from the 'surrogate parent', as well as have someone on hand to answer the questions he may not be able to ask you.

Later, write a summary of what you told your child, how

he reacted, the questions he asked and the support provided by the surrogate parent. Then post it to your former partner or his (her) legal representative. Keeping your former partner informed in all matters concerning your child is a form of insurance which pays dividends later in terms of your child's best interests.

3

Setting up a support structure

Life goes on. That cliché will be repeated to you more than any other through the difficult times ahead, by relatives, friends, counsellors and acquaintances trying to comfort you or snap you out of your despair. At times, you will resent it furiously, but eventually, it may become your own catch-cry, your morale booster as you marshal your resources to face up to the demands of the day. For, however the breakdown of your marriage affects your lifestyle, your standard of living, your values and your tenets for survival, you realise it hasn't, after all, brought about the end of the world—or even your world. The clock still ticks, the children still need to be fed, bathed and sent to school each day, a home has to be maintained . . . life goes on.

But, in the first few shaky days after the walk out, you may wonder how on earth you are going to cope. And, ironically, just when you most need people around you, you are likely to shut them out, close your doors, pretend all's well, in a vain attempt to 'keep up a front' because you believe that is what is expected of you.

If this is what you are doing, you are courting disaster. Even if you are emotionally strong, or independent enough, financially, to employ people to cushion you against some of life's sharp corners, there will surely come a time, sooner or later, when you are going to need help—either advice or simply someone to give you a hand when you are physically or emotionally exhausted. So why not start setting up a support structure for yourself and your child now, before things get on top of you . . . ?

There is a lot of truth in the old adage 'a problem shared is a problem halved'. This is not to suggest that you rush around crying on everyone's shoulder, but simply means that talking through your immediate reactions, your fears for the future, your financial worries and your plans for the next few days, weeks, months with *someone* will put things in their proper perspective and help you sort out your priorities. There is also the important consideration of the emotional release this affords you, especially if you can let yourself go completely, with a few outbursts of anger and tears which will undoubtedly be rewarded with a cup of tea, laced with lots of T.L.C. (tender, loving care)!

The key person in your support structure, if you are fortunate enough to have close family living near, will probably be your mother, or some other older female relative who can be available to you and your child, both as an emotional anchor and a surrogate mother when the need arises.

In the absence of family, a close friend could provide the shoulder you need to cry and lean on. If you are really on your own, you should make the effort to establish a link with one of the many voluntary crisis counselling set-ups now established in most communities. You can reach them via your local church, infant welfare centre, hospital or municipal offices. In some areas, crisis centres are listed in the emergency section of telephone directories to provide instant support as soon as you dial the number.

Even if you are surrounded by loving family and friends, it is still a good idea to tap in to an outside counselling set-up. As well as providing a sympathetic environment for you to air your fears and grievances, trained counsellors can offer something extra: objectivity. However intelligent, articulate and experienced family and friends might be, if they care about you they can't help being emotionally involved. Time spent with professional or trained voluntary advisers can provide the necessary balance to help you take your first, sure steps towards a secure, single life.

So don't wait for your problems to accumulate and overwhelm you. Get in touch with *someone* right away, with whom you can discuss your immediate and long term future, from what government benefits you might be entitled to, to how to buy food and pay bills until regular maintenance and child support payments are made, either by your former partner or as a government funded pension. (Some supporting custodian parents are afraid to reveal their problems to official welfare officers in case they have their children taken away from them and put into care. Custodian fathers are especially concerned that they risk being considered unfit to care for their children and still go out to work every day. Only rarely does this happen, and then a decision to remove children from the care of their remaining parent is usually based on the inability of the parent to care for them, due to mental or physical ill health or their obvious neglect. It is in the best interests of all concerned—the children, the parents and the government—to contribute to the emotional and financial support of one-parent families in their own homes rather than underwrite the whole cost of caring for them in government funded institutions.)

If you haven't already thought about seeking legal advice regarding your financial entitlement to joint family assets and the care, custody and control of your child, this is the time to do so. If you can afford the cost, you should make an appointment to see a solicitor of your own choosing. Otherwise, contact the Legal Aid Service for free legal advice and representation in court.

In practical terms, one of the first things you can do to earn respite from potential financial problems is to solicit the support of the people who control your family cash flow. Before you attempt to afford priority to any bills or demands for payment, find out exactly how much money you have or may be entitled to from joint holdings. To do this, begin by making an appointment to see your bank manager. A teller or even the chief accountant won't do. Only the manager has the authority to give you the information you need and the assurance of a temporary overdraft if you require one. Ask him to run a special check to see if there are any deposit accounts held in your partner's name that you may not know about, or any loan accounts for which you may be jointly responsible. Also, find out to what extent you may be liable. If you discover that you have been left with no funds, you may be able to secure a small overdraft against anticipated allowances, child support or pensions.

You should also make a thorough search of bureau drawers, files, old suitcases—anywhere you may have stored old papers pertaining to household administration—for any records of savings accounts, bonds, certificates of ownership of anything which might be regarded as accumulated negotiable assets. Even if you come across an old deposit savings book which has been inactive for years, it's worth telephoning the branch and asking if there are funds still in it.

If you find anything which could provide you with immediate funds, take it to your legal adviser so that he can negotiate its collection on your behalf, or arrange for you to receive your fair share of the proceeds jointly with your former partner. This goes for anything from jewellery to power tools, the family car to a lottery ticket.

Next, contact any local retailers to whom you may owe money; the grocer, the chemist, your newsagent. Explain the situation briefly and ask them to extend your credit for a limited period (you can determine this by finding out when your supportive pension or family payment will come through from the relevant authority). In most cases, especially if you are known, retailers are co-operative.

Now telephone any credit companies with whom you may have accounts, and make an appointment to see the respective credit managers. Tell them you need a period of grace, a breathing space of, say, two or three months, before you make another payment and they will probably be able to arrange deferment of payments. Most credit companies prefer to accept delayed payments to having to go through the legalities of repossessing goods or going through the courts for their money, but you must give them time to adjust their records.

In cases of hardship, in which custodian parents are left without warning or financial resources, emergency cash grants are sometimes made by government agencies to cover immediate necessities, such as food, electricity and gas bills, public transport fares, children's school lunches and so on. You can find out more about these emergency cash grants from your nearest government welfare or social services office.

Your health and the health of your child will play an important part in how you both cope in the months ahead. Even if you are fit and healthy now, see your family doctor and let him know what's going on at home. Knowledge of family relationships can give him significant insight into the cause of any symptoms of mental or physical ill health which may appear later on.

Just as doctors gain insight into the cause of symptoms of ill health through knowledge of a patient's family relationships and home environment, a child's teacher may be able to draw on that knowledge to make allowances for any changes in a pupil's achievement levels and behavioural pattern. This can help a child tremendously if he is having difficulty concentrating on his class work or mixing with his peers—common side effects of upheavals at home. So, it is absolutely necessary that you inform your child's class teacher, and possibly the school principal of the changes at home, and the related stress and anxieties which may be building up inside your child. When you consider that he spends more of his waking day at school than he does at home, it is not unreasonable to assume that his anxiety may manifest itself in irregular behaviour and attitudes at school. It helps your child, as well as your child's teachers, if you alert the staff to the possibility.

Parents often overlook the influence a teacher has over a child's emotional development, as well as his academic potential. But a good teacher can inspire a whole class with confidence and self esteem, and most welcome the opportunity to work on that aspect of their vocation with individual children in need of extra support. This is especially applicable at primary school level when the pupil-teacher relationship is closest.

At secondary school level, unless special attention is drawn to the problems a child may face at home, the rigours of adolescence and the pressures of school work experienced by most high school students may be held accountable for his (her) peculiar behaviour, and your child could be deprived of the understanding and help teachers may otherwise have been able to offer. Whatever your child's age, from kinder through secondary school, you should include his teachers in his support structure.

The parents of your child's closest friends could also be of great help to him if you enlist their support. It is never easy to air one's personal problems—however close the recipients of your family secrets might be—but this is the time to consider your child's long term interests above such temporary personal discomforts as embarrassment. (Your confidences will almost certainly be heard with sympathy and understanding—with the latest statistics for the number of one-parent families in the developed world put at more than one in three, it is highly likely they have experienced, or can expect to experience, similar problems themselves at some time . . .)

After-school group activity leaders should also be notified of your child's new single-parent status. The more people who regularly come into contact with him, who know, the better, if only to relieve him of the strain of trying to pretend nothing has changed.

Personal safety is another problem a single mother now has to consider, with no man in the house. There is little doubt that you are more vulnerable in your new situation than you were before, and for your own peace of mind, and that of your child, there are a few, simple precautions you can take to ensure your safety, as far as anyone can.

First, notify the police that you are living alone with your child. They may not run any special checks, but a call for help at a later date will have them on the spot and in the picture quicker if they have been alerted previously. You will also find the police can offer suggestions to make your home secure against unwelcome visitors. If your former partner's behaviour has prompted you to take out a restraining order, you should leave a copy of it at your local police station to give them the authority they need to take appropriate action if you feel threatened in the future.

Next, set up some sort of emergency procedure with a male relative or neighbourhood husband whom you can rely on to see you through bumps in the night, electrical failures and confrontations with persistent door-to-door salesmen. Just the knowledge that you can call someone can offset the fear at the time of the crisis, and will enable you to keep the whole thing in its proper perspective. It's also a comfort to a small child to know that Uncle Steve, or Uncle John will come over and fix the banging door or find out who is walking up the side path at night, if mummy can't handle it.

The men who make up your emergency support structure may also help you out with minor emergencies, like leaking taps, flat tyres, cold hot-water systems and fused electrical circuits—small irritations in themselves but which, tackled unsuccessfully alone, can reduce a grown woman (and a small child) to tears.

(*Custodian fathers* are probably well equipped to handle most personal safety and home maintenance crises themselves, but you may find you need help in other areas. A small child, for instance, may choke on his food, develop a rash, a high temperature, or some other symptoms a mother might normally be able to cope with, but are out of the range of your everyday experience. Thus, it makes sense to alert a female relative or a neighbourhood mother to the fact that you may need to call on her judgement or advice at some odd hour—these things always seem to happen late at night when your family doctor's surgery is closed, and the locum is already out on a call.

(You will also find your neighbourhood mothers are a valuable source of information about what to put in school lunches, whether or not to make your child eat his greens every night, and just how much soap powder you really need to wash your average five kilogram load. This can give you some good ideas for inexpensive nutritious family meals, too.)

But however hard you work at keeping your one-parent home and family running smoothly, however well you have structured your support system, and that of your child, there are going to be times when things fall apart or pile up on top of you so heavily that you feel you simply cannot carry on without a break from the constant pressure of your responsibilities. This is when you need a surrogate family for your child, with whom he can stay overnight, or for a weekend, or even a few days, while you take time out to rest and re-evaluate your priorities.

Family are the ideal surrogates, of course. Grandparents, aunts and uncles, the people your child knows and loves and feels comfortable with, and who would probably welcome him with open arms and cosset him with tender loving care while you wallow in a warm bath, dress up and go to a show or visit friends with whom you can talk as a person, not a parent.

Dismiss any nagging doubts you might have, as you toss another handful of mineral salts into the bathwater, or weep with laughter in the sixth row of the stalls, about letting your child down by ducking out of your parenting role for a few hours, or days—he is probably enjoying the break from you, too. It is all too easy to overlook a child's tension or boredom, because it is usually transmitted as bad behaviour, which instead of invoking sympathy from parents, usually triggers a chain reaction of equally bad behaviour or irritability. Just as you need a break now and then, so does your child, and this is especially true of older children from, say, ten years and over. It does them good to get away from the ever present problems associated with your separation and divorce plans, and the constant reminders of their own insecurity.

If you have no relatives or close friends with whom your child can stay, you might consider contacting your local welfare or community services officer who can, in turn, put you in touch with a voluntary emergency foster care group, made up of ordinary family units willing and able to take a child (or children, in the case of brothers and sisters) into their hearts and homes at a moment's notice, to relieve parents of their immediate responsibilities in the event of any sort of personal emergency. This sort of temporary emergency care in no way detracts from your regular capability as a custodian parent, so you don't need to worry unnecessarily about losing care and control of your child permanently as a result of taking a short break.

A secondary school aged child would benefit greatly from an organised school or activity group excursion, which at the same time, would give you a break too. Money may be tight, but if you can possibly afford it, send your child on any or all he may wish to take part in. (In cases of financial hardship, funds are available from the Departments of Education and community welfare services to cover the costs of school trips and other group excursions, so if you cannot find the money yourself, ask your child's school teacher or activity group leader to make inquiries on your behalf.)

Pets may also be used as props or an emotional escape valve for your child at this time. A cuddly cat or dog who gives and accepts your child's love unconditionally may fill at least part of the gap left in his capacity for the love exchange he enjoyed on a daily basis with his other, part-time parent. If you decide to provide this sort of comfort for your child, you must weigh the pros and cons very carefully before you commit your child—and yourself—to the responsibilities of caring for another living being.

First of all, any pets—cats, dogs, guinea pigs, hamsters, even goldfish—cost money to feed, equip and maintain in good health, and anyone on a limited budget has to take every outgoing cent into consideration.

If you feel you can afford the initial outlay and continued expense, you must now give thought to the time a pet takes up and the extra work it may cause you at a time when you may already be stretched to your limits. Pups and kittens look cute but they are, invariably, untrained, so be prepared to spend several minutes wiping up puddles at regular intervals throughout every day for about six weeks, or however long it takes for your pet to get the hang of controlling his movements or scratching at the door to be let out.

Also, unless you are very lucky, your cute little pup or kitten will probably have fleas, which, if you intend it to be a source of physical comfort to your child, you will want to remove as soon as possible—or regularly, depending on whether it comes into contact with other neighbourhood pets.

This can be a time-consuming, irritating chore, not for the squeamish.

There is also the need to fence off your garden adequately to ensure your child's new pet doesn't wander and get lost, or worse—run over. Unless you are prepared for all this, you could be setting your child up for yet another loss when you decide, however reluctantly, that you cannot cope with the added expense and extra work and give his pet away. (You can cut out the drudgery of house-training a pet by choosing a young adult cat or dog. There is a bonus in this approach to pet hunting, too, in that you get a good idea of the character and intelligence of the dog and how it would fit into the family and the facilities available to it.)

In the final analysis, you may decide it will be better for you and subsequently for your child, to buy a new, soft, cuddly toy dog, cat, bear or whatever, which can be cuddled and crooned to, cried on and occasionally punched up without fear of the live consequences of puddles, scratches and bites.

4

Guilt—yours and your child's

Next to jealousy, guilt is regarded by many family therapists as the most self destructive emotion the human mind can harbour. Left unchecked, it feeds upon itself and can seriously incapacitate a person mentally and even physically, manifesting itself as withdrawal or violence, with all the stops in between.

Guilt is one of the most common and enduring reactions to marriage breakdown, whoever the 'guilty' partner may be—husband or wife, the one who walks out or the one who stays. And the guilt factor plays a significant part in everyone's behaviour, not only that of the partners to each other but the interaction between parents and child, child and siblings or peers.

Some parents understand this, and try to come to terms with the guilt factor, making allowances for occasional outbursts of irrational behaviour in themselves, their children and their former partners. Others try merely to compensate for it by heaping material rewards on their former partners, and especially their children, to counterbalance their guilt. A good number give in to guilt—deserved or not—and allow it to stunt their emotional growth and subsequently, that of their children. Most parents, however concerned and aware they may be about their children's welfare and healthy emotional development, overlook entirely the guilt factor experienced and contributed by their children. Unchecked, the burden of a child's guilt (albeit unfounded) can have the most tragic consequences of all.

Here we look at the most common reactions to guilt during the separation-divorce trauma—and how to avoid them—through the actual experiences of men, women and children who were unable to cope with the effects.

Jane is thirty-two and the mother of a six-year-old daughter. She and her husband, Gary, were married for five years before their daughter was born, and until then had enjoyed a carefree existence on a dual income, travelling extensively and sampling the sophisticated pleasures of Sydney's more expensive night spots.

With the birth of her daughter, Jane was forced to curtail her outside activities in the interests of being a good mother (by her own reckoning). She gave up her job which affected the couple's income and limited the amount she had to spend on herself by way of clothes and accessories, and became, by her own comparison, dull and 'mumsy'.

But she enjoyed her new role, and adored her child. The fact that her husband had not compromised his lifestyle to fit into the new pattern their daughter had created for them did not worry her unduly. She felt, given time, that her husband would settle down, too. So sure was Jane about this that she pressed Gary for another child. The prospect of doubling their domestic commitment, as Gary saw it, triggered the inevitable. The marriage broke down and Gary moved into a bachelor flat, opting out of all commitment to Jane and their daughter except their financial support.

Jane was left with a daughter with no father, and a staggering burden of guilt for having—as she saw it—driven the child's father away by neglecting his needs in favour of her own. Her guilt was further reinforced by Gary's ready acceptance of his financial responsibilities to Jane and their daughter. Finally, faced with the continual reminder of her guilt—her daughter—Jane came to loathe the child she loved, and eventually rejected her.

Patient probing by a psychiatrist, after Jane had attempted to abandon her little girl outside a supermarket, brought her back to the point at which her initial guilt—at this stage, a perfectly natural reaction—had been allowed to grow out of control until it had obscured the truth. The real reason that the marriage had broken down was not because Jane had pushed Gary into a commitment he could not make, it was simply that Gary could not make a commitment to the sort of marriage Jane wanted. Had Jane been objective enough about her guilt reaction in its initial stages, she might have seen the weakness in her marriage—and her husband—and been able to build a firmer future for herself and her daughter, with a more positive attitude . . .

Kay had been married for just three years when she decided to take her two year old daughter and eleven month old son away from the home they shared with her husband, Bill, and seek a divorce. Although Bill was an alcoholic and had inflicted several severe beatings on his wife and threatened their children, Kay allowed herself to accept the burden of guilt for the actual break-up and the subsequent one parent status of her children.

Her guilt was fed by Bill who claimed he only drank because Kay made him feel inadequate as a lover and a provider. It was reinforced by Bill's mother who told Kay that all Bill really needed to become a responsible husband and father was loving support and a little more understanding.

Against the advice of her parents, her family doctor (who had treated Kay for multiple bruises and lacerations on several occasions), and their few, close friends, Kay gave in to her guilt and went back to Bill to give the marriage another go.

Some three months later, after bill had consumed a considerable quantity of wine and spirits, the couple went to bed and Bill began to make love to Kay. Before she could respond, the baby cried, and Kay moved automatically to get out of bed and tend her child. Unable to tolerate her 'rejection' of him in his irrational, drunken state, Bill struck Kay first, and then the baby, to 'make it shut up'.

Now Kay and the children are once more living with her parents, and awaiting a divorce. Although the bruises have faded and the split lips have healed, both Kay and her son—and her two year old daughter who witnessed their ordeal—will probably bear the emotional scars of the consequences of Kay's misplaced guilt for the rest of their lives.

Had Kay listened to the advice of her parents, her doctor and friends, who were able to assess the reasons for the marriage breakdown and the risks she would run in the event of a reconciliation more objectively than she could, Kay might have seen Bill for what he really was, and been able to reverse Bill's mother's loaded opinion.

Instead of assuming the guilt for calling a halt to the marriage, she could have turned her reaction round to assuming responsibility for calling a halt to Bill's behaviour. If she still felt any lingering guilt, she might have given Bill the hope of a reconciliation, conditional upon his complete recovery from dependence on alcohol. Help from professional therapists would have given him the chance to put her rejection of him as a lover in its proper perspective, enabling him to keep a job, and thus become an adequate provider.

Julie is forty-two and happily married to a man some years her junior. She has two children, now grown and living away from home, by a former marriage, who get along wonderfully well with their stepfather and are delighted at their mother's new found happiness.

But there is a cloud on Julie's bright horizon . . . she cannot have a child with the man she loves to make their happiness complete. For Julie allowed the burden of guilt to weigh too heavily and too long in the years after the breakdown of her first marriage and subsequent divorce.

Julie was twenty when her first child was born, twenty-two when the second one came along. At first, her (then) husband, John, and their two little girls took up almost all of Julie's time and interest, but gradually she came to realise that something was missing in her life. She felt unfulfilled as a person, wanted more from life than achievement based on servicing the needs of other people.

Before her early marriage, Julie had finished high school and gained university entrance in her final examinations. Against John's wishes, after her younger child was weaned, Julie resumed her education on a part-time basis, and eventually earned a teaching qualification which enabled her to boost the family's income and fill a void in terms of her own personal achievement.

But, as soon as Julie started teaching, things went wrong between her and John. He felt that a wife's place was in the home, offering comfort to all who came in, whenever they came in, and resented Julie's obvious pleasure at being able to serve a useful purpose elsewhere. The more enthusiasm she expressed for her job, the less co-operative he became, refusing, eventually, to do anything about the house to facilitate Julie's early start, or preparation for the following day's teaching.

Eventually, their relationship disintegrated altogether, and John left Julie for a widow with two small boys who wanted nothing more from life than a home with a husband in it. John and Julie met frequently, through the years that followed, their relationship with each other friendly, their mutual concern for their children the only thing they really had in common. But as Julie watched her children grow up disadvantaged (by her comparison with the other children of two-parent families who lived around them), she held her own ambitions responsible for the fact that her girls were fatherless.

So dedicated did she become to compensating for the loss of a father, that Julie spent all her spare time with her daughters, or sewing them beautiful clothes, or planning special treats, and allocated no time for herself to meet new partners, or form new relationships.

It wasn't until her girls were grown and forming relationships of their own leaving no time for Julie, that she realised what a waste of time her long, lonely guilt trip had been. By the time she met Ray she felt she could not run the risks involved in having a late baby. With the wisdom of hindsight, she knew that she had overlooked the basic ingredient of her marriage breakdown all those years ago: she and John were incompatible from the beginning, neither one of them was 'guilty' of wrecking the marriage . . .

Paul had a different problem. In his opinion, he really was guilty of wrecking his marriage. He didn't do it deliberately, but on reflection, he realised he might as well have done. When he married Sandra, he thought she was the loveliest, sexiest girl in the world and she had the same opinion of him. The trouble was that while Paul's opinion of Sandra was all that really mattered to her, Paul needed constant reassurance of his own 'worth' from other women as well as Sandra.

After a year or so, the happy couple decided to start a family. They were both in their late twenties and had no money worries due to Paul's high income and sales commissions, so there seemed no reason to wait. When Sandra was six months pregnant, she gave up her public relations job and put her creative energies to work making herself and their home as attractive as she could for Paul.

The hurt she suffered when she learned of Paul's affairs which he'd covered with excuses that he was working late at the office, almost overshadowed her joy at the birth of their daughter a few days later. But what put the marriage beyond repair was Paul's explanation of his escapades, when she came home from hospital. He told her, simply, that they 'didn't mean a thing'. It was his lack of commitment to their relationship that spelled separation and divorce for Sandra, and caused Paul to indulge himself in his guilt to the extent of ruining his second marriage, too.

The only way Paul could cope with the divorce and what he had done to cause it, was to shut himself off completely from Sandra and their infant daughter. And, although he never really recovered from the loss, he eventually found comfort in the arms of someone else. By the time he made the decision to marry her, he had matured to the point where he no longer needed constant reassurance from casual affairs and felt he could make a lasting commitment to his new wife.

The happiness he found with her was enhanced, some months later, by the news that she was expecting a baby. But for Paul, it couldn't last. The heavy mantle of guilt he had worn for so long because of his treatment of his first wife and child smothered the happiness he had found with his new wife and child. By the time the baby was born, Paul had reached the stage at which he could not love it without feeling he was betraying his first child. His guilt spilled over into his relationship with his second wife whom he finally turned on for trying, in his opinion, to usurp the position Sandra still rightfully held. And that marriage, too, ended in divorce.

Had Paul paused, between marriages, to consider how he might put his guilt to good use, instead of secreting it, like a wardrobe drinker, he might have turned it into a positive learning experience which could have enriched his second marriage and encompassed the lives of his first wife and child.

If he had accepted his guilt for what it was—the consequences of his earlier immaturity rather than deliberate cruelty—he could have enjoyed his new found happiness, and played a supportive role in the lives of Sandra and their child, all at the same time . . .

Greg was too young, really, even to know there was such a word as guilt, but he had a feeling for it, all the same. Greg's father had left home three days after his eighth birthday. Greg knew the date and remembered it exactly, because that was when he wished it would happen. He had left his new birthday bike out in the rain overnight, and his father had locked it in the garage for a week to teach him to look after it.

He'd heard the row from his bedroom, the night his father slammed out. It had been going on all evening, ever since his mother protested that a week was really too long. As his parents' voices reached an angry crescendo, Greg whispered the fateful words under his breath: 'I wish he'd go away and never come back . . . ' As soon as he heard the door bang shut, he had tried to take his wish back. He prayed to God until he fell asleep that he would never, ever, leave his bike out again if only his dad would come back. But his father stayed away.

As the weeks wore on, Greg realised how unhappy his mother was and this added to his guilt. After all, he had wished his father would go, hadn't he? He thought of owning up to his mother but then thought that she might be so angry that she would leave him, too, and then he would have no one. He would just have to work out a way to get his dad back by himself . . .

So committed did Greg become to his project to get his father to return that he lost interest in his school work, his food, his friends and his home life. He lost weight and, to his added shame, began to wet the bed. His mother called it 'withdrawal' when she took him to the family doctor. The psychiatrist to whom the doctor referred Greg spent several months coaxing the boy's guilty secret from him. It took just an hour with his mother and father together in the psychiatrist's consulting room to convince Greg that he wasn't to blame for the breakdown of his parents' marriage. Had they not considered him too young (or had they considered him in real terms, at all), they might have given him a reason when the walk out occurred, instead of leaving their child to search his own conscience for an answer that wasn't there . . .

The guilt an older child assumes for the responsibility of his parents' failed marriage can be just as devastating and equally undeserved. One of the new 'causes' of marital tension and eventual breakdown offered by middle-aged parents is the inability of their teenage children to get jobs. Mark was one such unemployed teenager. He had left school at sixteen with high hopes of following in his elder brother's footsteps by working for a couple of years to earn the money to go overseas. But Mark's brother had left school four years earlier, when jobs were easier to come by, and Mark found himself sitting at home all day, instead of working.

He didn't mind so much at first, when he still had hope. Each day he would get the papers then spend all morning going through them and phoning for interviews. But, as the number of jobs dwindled, so did Mark's hope. As the days wore on and became weeks and months, depression set in and Mark started sleeping in, sometimes until well after lunch. What, after all, was there to get up for?

It was then that things began to get really bad between his parents. They had never been what you'd call sweet, as far back as Mark could remember, but now the rows were going on non-stop, and somehow, they always seemed to centre around him. If the place wasn't tidy enough to suit dad when he came home at night, it was because mum couldn't clean properly with *him* home all day; if the tools were left all over the garage, what else could you expect with *him* hanging around in there with nothing else to do all day. Then there would be the back-and-forth rows . . . dad would call Mark a lazy so-and-so for not getting out and looking for a job, and mum would defend him, saying there were no jobs to get out and look for; mum would ask Mark to help with the household chores and dad would yell her out for trying to get him to do woman's work. But the worst rows erupted when Mark tried to buy into his parents' differences. Sometimes, he would try to get them to see each other's point of view, other times he was just so bored it was worth risking the consequences. And the consequences were that they would both turn on him!

Eventually, Mark's father cleared out and went to live with his secretary, a woman about the same age as Mark's mother but with no children. Although his mother never actually put her accusations into words, Mark felt that the blame was his all the same, and made the only decision he could if his parents were ever to get back together again—he left home.

As it turned out, Mark's parents didn't get back together again, because, of course, Mark was only the catalyst, not the cause of their marriage breakdown. The marriage had been deteriorating for some years, with neither partner willing to make the break and appear the 'baddie' to their children. The irritations caused by Mark's continual presence which upset his mother's routine and his father's peace of mind only served to open up the bigger issues which would probably have come to the surface sooner or later, anyway.

But no one could find Mark to explain all this to him. For the next eight months, he drifted from one refuge to another, sometimes it would be a friend's place, another time some charity house, more often the back of a mate's car. A parole officer was eventually assigned to Mark after he had been caught stealing to support his growing dependence on alcohol and drugs. The officer tried to convince Mark that his parents' problems were their own, not his, but by then his guilt was too deeply ingrained for even heroin, let alone a stranger, to erase.

The symptoms of guilt in children often go unrecognised because it is undeserved, so parents are not looking for it. But it may be useful to watch for such warning signals as irritability, tearfulness, violence (breaking toys, deliberately smashing a bike into a wall, slapping siblings or peers) and withdrawal. They are all indicative of frustration which could be the result of not being able to cope with imagined guilt.

Adult guilt left unturned can manifest itself in even more serious behavioural patterns resulting in dependence on legal and illegal drugs, alcoholism and physical violence, including child abuse by either the custodian or access parent.

Whatever the degree of guilt you may be carrying for your part in the breakdown of your marriage, the best thing you can do for your child's sake, as well as your own, is to make what amends you feel are necessary in a positive, supportive way, determine not to repeat your mistakes, and then put your guilty feelings out of your mind for good.

5

Discipline (tough love)

One of the basic requirements for survival for separated and divorced custodian parents is that they remain in control of what is left of the family unit. And yet, due to diminished emotional and sometimes physical capability, brought about by their own reaction to the stress and anxiety caused by the situation in which they find themselves, this is the time they are most likely to lose control, let go, give the unpopular side of parenting away.

The results of an over-relaxed attitude to discipline are rarely rewarding. In the short term, your child may appear to love you more if he's allowed to dip into the lolly jar whenever he wishes, or hang out at the pin-ball parlour until he chooses to come home, but in the long run his love may turn to contempt.

For all children, from infants to adolescents, need the constant reaffirmation of a parent's love and concern for them as expressed through reinforcing the boundaries of everyday discipline.

This is not to say that the separation-divorce period is the time to come down on your child with a crunch, tighten up, stay on top at all costs. Indeed, you will now be required to dispense discipline with far more sensitivity and flexibility than ever before, as you will have to take into consideration the see-saw balance of your child's emotional reactions to the structural changes brought about by separation and divorce, his anger and frustration at his inability to change things back as they were, and his occasional desire to pay back or punish both parents for causing him so much upheaval and unhappiness.

Nevertheless, the established rules and regulations of his immediate environment can provide him with the basic stability he desperately needs now and in the difficult months ahead. So, the aim of this chapter is to help parents—access as well as custodian—to *maintain* the standards normally required to facilitate harmonious interaction between the most important members of a child's world—himself, his mother and his father—while at the same time, recognising that due to the abnormal circumstances, some adjustments and allowances will have to be made.

Discipline is a complicated issue even in a two-parent family, but in the event of separation and divorce, one has to consider the problems of back-up support and follow-through brought about by the dispensers of discipline and authority living apart. Whereas before discipline and authority came from a combined source, straight down to your child, he is now placed at the bottom of an inverted triangle with two equi-distant power bases above him.

If your child is to have any chance of maintaining regular standards for himself and, consequently, some degree of peace of mind, it is obviously important that both parents set similar standards, endeavouring to put aside their differences and work together to achieve the continuity of love and authority which is absolutely essential to effective discipline.

Regrettably, the opposite more often occurs, with one or both parents attempting to manipulate or pay back the other by vying for the lion's share of their child's affection and admiration (however temporary) through, at best, over indulgence, at worst, flagrant disregard for the basic ground rules necessary for the child's mental and physical wellbeing. The end result of either of these attitudes is, of course, confusion for the child and, quite possibly, rejection of one or both parents. In either case, the child is the loser.

There are also vast differences in the interpretation of discipline in regard to a child's age, intelligence, comprehension and the significant influence of his peers. What applies to a pre-schooler doesn't work with an adolescent—that, at least, is usually understood. But what is often overlooked, especially by an access parent who may not be in continual touch with his (her) child's emotional and physical growth, is that subtle developments are constantly taking place which require constant reappraisal of a parent's attitudes towards discipline and authority. And, in the case of a child of separated or divorced parents, there may also be a basic resistance to any form of authority, born of disillusionment with the way authority—in a child's eyes his parent(s)—is behaving, all too often invoking the do-as-I-say-not-as-I-do amendment.

Your health—mental and physical—and that of your child will also have a profound effect upon the interaction between you, and the need for, and results of, discipline. There is little doubt that neither of you will be as emotionally stable now, or for some time to come, as you might have been in a 'normal', two-parent family situation, and the physical symptoms of anxiety and stress can leave both adults and children vulnerable and hostile.

Your family's diet, which you may have neglected with so many other things requiring your attention, has a tremendous bearing on your health in general and the fatigue factor in particular. Fatigue, whether it is the result of inadequate diet, increased physical exertion or lack of sleep, due to anxiety and stress, often manifests itself in unreasonable irritability and irrational behaviour in adults and children alike—neither of which traits is conducive to harmony in the home.

With all these aspects to consider, from the points of view of the custodian parent, the access parent and the child, it is easier to tackle the problems of discipline for the child of separated or divorced parents in three parts, always bearing in mind, of course, that each interacts with the other and must be considered as part of your whole approach if your child is to benefit from your attempts to provide emotional stability through reasonable discipline—reinforced, it should be remembered with oral and physical statements of love.

In the following pages, custodian and access parents will find case histories involving children in pre-school, primary school and high school age groups. These are provided as a basis of comparison with your own child's behaviour. Conclusions and information regarding attitudes, reactions to specific situations, health and future relationships are provided by behavioural experts and medical specialists.

1. Discipline in the custodian parent's home

The sort of situation which arises frequently with pre-schoolers who are unable to identify their emotions or anxieties and translate them into words with which to explain them and ask for reassurance, may best be illustrated by the following scenario, with you in the lead role . . .

It is late in the day, you have a million things on your mind, your head throbs intolerably, and little Johnny is banging a saucepan against the stove repeatedly, despite the fact you've asked him to stop at least three times. If your logic were not clouded by the traumatic events of separation and divorce, you would probably see the situation for what it really is: an entirely predictable, ritual stand-off common to two-year-olds and mothers under stress.

Had little Johnny banged the saucepan against the stove a month ago, when you were both feeling relatively secure, you might have told him to stop, once, then removed the pan from his hands with a verbal admonition. Now, under extreme pressure, you react by snatching the pan away and slapping Johnny smartly—not so much for what he has done but how it affected you. Little Johnny, on the other hand, surprised by your unusually explosive reaction reacts explosively himself, yelling and slapping at you. How you take it from here may set the pattern for weeks or months ahead.

You may grab the spatula and show him who is boss . . . or you might fall, sobbing, into the nearest chair, your hands over your ears and defeat in your eyes. Either way, you would lose control of little Johnny and your relationship with him for some time to come.

Ideally, you will walk out of the room and into your bedroom, the garden or some other quiet place where you can spend a few moments alone getting your emotions under control. In that time, you will evaluate the situation for what it is: over reaction on your part and subsequently Johnny's, supercharged to flashpoint by the build-up of tension over the breakdown of the marriage, in your case, and the mysterious disappearance of a father, in his.

Now you go back into the kitchen and take the pan from Johnny's hands, explaining as calmly as possible that he's making too much noise, might dent the stove, wake the baby or whatever. At the same time, devise some five minute project you can both share which pays a double dividend: it takes Johnny's mind off the rewarding noise the saucepan makes and by the attention you are giving him, reassures him of your love—which was probably all he really wanted in the first place and you were too preoccupied to notice.

Other symptoms of a pre-schooler's dissatisfaction, distress, frustration or anxiety which manifest themselves as 'bad behaviour' include temper tantrums with all the trimmings (body stiffening, breath holding, screaming), spitting, biting, reverting to the bottle (especially if there is a younger sibling), bed wetting, pants soiling, toy smashing and doll bashing.

While some sort of disciplinary action is usually required if you want your child to mature into a tolerable adult, care should be taken not to mete out punishment in accordance with your own reaction. In other words, judge the 'offence' on its own merits, not by the amount of irritation it causes you. In most cases, simply answering the plea behind your child's behaviour, followed by rational action to prevent the incident recurring, works better than verbal or physical abuse.

With older, primary school children, the symptoms of insecurity and frustration may be directed at you in a more positive manner. Although they need reassurance of their parents' love every bit as much as pre-schoolers do, it may seem, at times, as if they are trying to achieve the opposite, as shown in the following example . . .

You are sitting, having a few tears, in the armchair in the living room. All you want is a few minutes time to yourself, to let go a little, unwind . . . Suzie, eight, turns the TV up and down, up and down. You get up and walk into the kitchen. Suzie follows, and deliberately opens and shuts, opens and shuts the refrigerator door. You look at her and read the challenge in her eyes—she might as well ask, literally, what you are going to do about it.

The answer is, you have two choices. You can scream, slap, and slam out . . . or you can withdraw, firmly, and think the situation through until you come up with the cause of Suzie's unreasonable behaviour, before you take her to task for it. And the cause is, of course, her concern at your unhappiness. She is worried and frustrated because she cannot understand why you are crying. Her eight year old's logic works this way: by diverting your attention from whatever it is that is upsetting you, by whatever means at her disposal (and at eight, they are limited), Suzie can possibly stop you crying. More important, perhaps, she can find out whether or not it is her fault you are crying. So concerned is she at your unhappiness and the possibility that she may have caused it, that she is willing to pay the price of punishment if she can change your mood to something she can understand and accept—even anger.

You can prevent a showdown by letting Suzie know you are reading the more important of the two conflicting messages she is sending out. Give her your attention long enough to explain the real reason for your tears (maybe not the *whole* reason but enough to exonerate her from any blame) and then ask her if she could possibly cheer you up. Ten to one she'll stick out her tongue, but it will probably have the desired effect and you will both have learned something about each other and ended up friends, instead of enemies.

Shouting, swearing and fighting, generally directed at siblings and peers are also outward signs of inner turmoil among primary school children. 'I hate you!' yelled at peers or parents is often an eight, nine or ten-year-old's way of saying 'I don't understand why you've got two parents and I've got one' or 'I don't understand why you are splitting up and making me unhappy'.

Yelling back at a child who has reached screaming point hardly ever has a positive effect. It answers none of his questions, quiets none of his fears. While it may be difficult for you, in your own over-emotional state, to summon the self control to be calm and reasonable, as an adult, you should have the edge on your child in the area of self control, so use it now. Deal with his aggression as if it were some physical symptom that all is not well, one you could find more sympathy for, like a headache or a sore throat. See what you can do to take away the pain, then go to work on the cause. You may not achieve a cure overnight, but constant treatment—regular doses of time and attention, and simple TLC—can restore his behavioural pattern to normal.

Adolescents may well have a harder time than their younger brothers and sisters coping with their parents' separation and divorce. Not only do they have to handle the structural changes around them but also the physiological changes of their own bodies.

It is difficult for parents, too, to distinguish between normal boundary testing prevalent among teenagers trying to assert their burgeoning independence, and reactionary behaviour born of resentment and frustration at the behaviour of their parents. There is also the double disillusionment of teenagers and their parents for letting each other down just when they need each other most.

Generally speaking, in this situation, a teenager may react by pushing his (her) parents to the limit of their endurance in an all out effort to solicit their support even at the risk of severe restrictions or similar punitive measures. Parents, on the other hand, often react to the challenge by cracking down on their sons and daughters to such an extent that they rob them of the right to reason, or let go completely, leaving their children to drift helplessly until they are out of sight of their moorings altogether.

In the case of one sixteen year old boy, whose separated parents took the easy way out and let him go his own way, the results were irreversible . . .

Steve started playing up the night after his father left. He'd had things explained to him . . . how his parents had come to a mutual understanding to separate. His father had left to move in with a girl who worked in his office and he hoped, in time, Steve would visit them, come to regard their home as his, and so on. His mother seemed to be happy with the new arrangement. Resigned might have been a better description of her attitude, but Steve had not yet learned to discern the difference; to him it seemed everyone was happy—except him. But no one bothered to find out how he felt about the break-up, before or after it happened. They obviously didn't give a damn. Okay! He wouldn't give a damn about them, either. He'd go his own sweet way, too . . . he'd show them!

He spent that night at a friend's house, without bothering to phone home and let his mother know where he was. The following morning, he strolled into his own home and without a word of explanation walked straight past his father, who had returned home at his mother's request to deal with Steve's disappearance. His mother had taken a sedative and was sleeping. He still didn't say a word when his father roared him out for causing so much trouble, and finally slammed out back to his new home. He simply helped himself to one of his mother's tranquillisers and went along to his room.

He repeated the exercise a week or so later, but now he came home decidedly hung over and collapsed on the couch. This time, his father didn't wait to give him hell; he'd left by the time Steve woke up. And his mother, as usual, was sleeping in.

On subsequent occasions when Steve stayed out all night and got drunk, his parents reacted with diminishing interest. Eventually, Steve stayed out more than he came home at night, which seemed to excite no interest at all on the part of either parent. It finally interested the police, who came across him lying in a coma, in the back of an old car, where his mates had left him after an all night party, to sleep off the combined effects of alcohol and his mother's tranquillisers. By then, it was too late for his parents to react at all—Steve died the following day . . .

Not all adolescents contending with the dual burden of their own physiological and sociological changes, plus the structural changes of their parents' separation and divorce, turn to alcohol and drugs or stay out all night. But you may experience lesser symptoms of their insecurity, such as staying out late, exaggerated dress and mannerisms, a tendency to gravitate towards their aggressively sexual peers.

Ironically, although your adolescent may want to talk to you about his insecurity, and you may want to ease him (her) through this difficult period, your own unfamiliar behaviour during the separation-divorce trauma may set you apart. If you feel this might be the case, you may find it helpful to recruit the services of an advocate through whom you can communicate with each other. A sympathetic grandparent, a trusted relative, a youth worker or school teacher may be more successful at putting across your concern for your child and your need for his help, and vice versa, at least, in the initial stages. Once *détente* has been re-established, you should encourage regular discussions about each other's problems to keep the lines of communication open. If you are talking, you probably won't be fighting—you may even discover you have a lot in common with both of you preparing for independent lives.

2. Discipline in the access parent's home

Unlike a custodian parent, an access parent cannot practise discipline—or love, which is the counterbalance that keeps discipline in perspective—with any real degree of continuity, because he (she) cannot be with their child on a continuous basis. Thus, there cannot be the daily give and take, the mini-rows and abortive flare-ups which allow a regular parent to practise discipline on a sliding scale that tempers the top end with familiarity. Consequently, an access parent has a tendency to either overkill or overlook when it comes to selecting the right reaction to his visiting child's unreasonable behaviour. And there is little doubt that unless an access parent is extremely watchful of his own emotions, resentment of his former partner may cloud the issue and his reaction to it. The following true-life drama, with you in the leading role, may serve to illustrate this important aspect of discipline in the access parent's home . . .

Paul, aged three, is sitting on the cold, tiled floor of one of our better known, fast food family restaurants, immediately in front of the take-away counter. The crowd is edging closer, eager to place orders, but Paul refuses to move, despite all your patient reasoning or whispered threats, unless you agree to allow him to carry his own order out to the car. He stacks his case by putting it in an aggressively shrill voice which ensures you are the centre of attention. The other customers are obviously interested to see who wins.

You try walking off and leaving him to follow, but all he does is lie down and beat his heels against the floor. You return to pick him up with your one free arm and he arches his back, stiffens his body and kicks you in the knees, stomach and chest. 'Mummy lets me', he cries, over and over again.

At this stage, you are faced with three choices. You can capitulate and let him carry out his burger, fries and thick shake, or you can whack him a good one on the seat of his jeans to let him know you are still on top. Either way, the result will be an *impasse* because, in his excited state, Paul would now probably drop the lot, and if you whack him, will almost certainly be crying too hard to eat—which was, after all the object of the exercise. Or, you could compromise . . . but first you will have to withdraw, regroup your own emotions, and set about repairing his.

Your first move should be to retire to the nearest table and put down your order. Now, while you are waiting for Paul to tire of his performance (which he will, quite quickly with no audience), consider the cause of all the overreaction—yours and his. The clue is in what he said, over and over at the beginning of the debacle, 'Mummy lets me . . . '

All that Paul really wanted to do was assert his new-found independence, show off his newly acquired skill, to you. And, if you are honest with yourself, you were probably over-reacting to your own irritability at not being able to be around Paul enough, in your new role as access parent, to notice his gradual acquisition of new skills, and the fact that his mother—as custodian parent—is. Or maybe you were embarrassed at the attention your lack of judgement earned you from the other customers. Anyway, by the time you've thought it through, Paul will have wandered up to your table and started on his fries. This is the time to offer him *something* to carry out to the car . . .

When considering the cause, effect and possible punishment of unreasonable behaviour in pre-schoolers, access parents should always bear in mind the unsettling effect of change on most small children.

Any change to a pre-schooler's environment, food, clothing (even to what he takes off or puts on first), toileting, bed-time or any other facet of his regular routine, can result in very real feelings of insecurity, which in turn can result in the sort of behavioural displays listed in part one of this chapter dealing with behavioural changes between custodian parents and pre-schoolers.

Prevention is always better than punishment and the most effective way to deal with discipline is to reduce the need for it. The best way an access parent of a pre-schooler can do this is to ask the custodian parent for regular, updated information about your child's preferences, new skills and areas in which he still needs help, or problems which may have developed since you last spent time with him.

Children of primary school age are just as vulnerable as pre-schoolers when they are on unfamiliar ground. Their insecurity often shows up as aggression, excessively high spirits and constant demands for attention. It is difficult, sometimes, to remember this when you are on unfamiliar ground yourself, playing the mother as well as the father role if you have your child to stay overnight with you. The following case history shows the sort of mistakes that can occur if an access parent misinterprets his child's desperate pleas for reassurance as wilful disobedience.

Emma was seven when her parents separated. As an only child, she had developed a very close bond with her mother, which grew even closer when her father, David, left the family home. But David loved Emma, too, and wanted to continue his father role in the fullest possible sense. So he applied for, and was granted a one-in-four weekends access ruling which required Emma to spend her first night ever away from her mother.

As her first day in her father's flat drew to a close, Emma became fractious and demanding, irritating David to such an extent that he told her, angrily, to get ready for bed. Emma reacted by running to her room, sobbing for her mother. David followed and tried to help her into her nightclothes but his little daughter responded by shouting at him to get out.

Ready for bed at last, her tears all but dried, Emma came out of her room and demanded a drink. David gave her one. Five minutes later, she wanted a biscuit. She got that, too. A little while later, Emma was out of her room again, wanting another drink, but this time David told her, firmly to get back into bed. From then on, for the next hour, Emma kept up a constant barrage of noisy demands—for food, drinks, to get up and watch TV, for more books, her coloured pencils, anything which might bring David back into her room, or get her out of it. At last, David did go back to her room—to turn out her light.

But David didn't know that his daughter had developed an overwhelming fear of the dark since he had left the family home (a psychiatrist told him later it may have had something to do with the fact that he had left at night, while Emma was asleep). He turned a deaf ear to her insistent demands that he return once more and turn it back on. He felt sure she'd settle down eventually, stop crying and go to sleep.

Emma did, eventually, stop crying. She almost stopped breathing, too, as she began to experience her first asthma attack. It was only because David tip-toed back to her room, to temper his discipline with a goodnight kiss, that he discovered Emma's distress. The doctor he called relieved the child's symptoms for that night, but David still blames himself, rightly or wrongly, for the recurring attacks that Emma, now nine, still has.

In the case of older children, boredom is often the cause of unreasonable behaviour which can lead to a stand-off situation with either parent, custodian or access. In the custodial home, an adolescent is likely to get bored and resentful when he (she) misses the companionship he once shared with his now absent parent. In the access parent's home, he is more likely to be bored with nothing familiar to hand, nowhere familiar to go and no one familiar to 'rap' with, once the novelty of a new stereo has worn off and news has been exchanged with the access parent.

The usual symptoms of adolescent boredom—exaggerated indolence, sloppy eating habits, excessive noise, 'dumb' insolence—can rarely be relieved by disciplinary action, ultimatums or adult sarcasm (a popular substitute for corporal punishment employed by parents when dealing with children too big to slap). The only really effective action you can take to combat the effects of adolescent boredom is to toss it right back to your child and ask him (her) what he'd like to do or where he'd like to go.

If you sense that the reasons behind your child's unacceptable behaviour could lie deeper than boredom, you might handle it better if you try to bring them out into the open. You can do this by encouraging your child to open up, discuss whatever might be bugging him, or talking to your former partner, your child's teacher or school counsellor.

3. The health factor—yours and your child's

The separation-divorce trauma can have a seriously debilitating effect on the physical well-being, as well as the emotional state of all concerned—a factor which is often overlooked when considering behavioural attitudes and exchanges between parents and children in this situation. But medical research has proved that if you are feeling under par you are more inclined to overreact to comparatively trivial irritations. And this is the time, due to the million and one other things on your mind, you are least likely to look after yourself physically.

Whether you feel unwell or not, you should make an appointment with your family doctor to put him in the picture regarding any stress or anxiety you or your child may be experiencing as a result of your domestic upheaval. It's a good idea to have him check you for anaemia (a common cause of fatigue among women) and high blood pressure (common symptom of stress among men). Tell him about any headaches, high temperatures, persistent coughs or digestive upsets you or your child may have had recently. This is not the time to suppress these sort of symptoms with self prescribed analgesics.

Now, turn your attention to your diet. Health food fads aside, how we feel depends to a very great extent on what we eat. The right food is an important preventative of poor health. It can also relieve some of the more common complaints, notably fatigue, which can have a significant affect on family relationships.

Custodian parents are most at risk in the area of inadequate diet. Although they may attend to the dietary needs of their children most diligently, they often skip meals altogether themselves, to save money or simply because they cannot be bothered to eat. If you are skipping meals to save money, you are practising a false economy. From the money you save you must subtract the cost of increased expenditure on cigarettes, sweets, patent medicines, the odd, self-indulgent cream bun, or, if you really let yourself run down, doctor's bills. If you are missing meals because you cannot be bothered to eat, you are putting your child as well as yourself at risk, because sooner or later, you are going to get really sick, and then who will look after him? In either case, the spin-off for your child will be your increased irritability and inability to deal with his problems as well as your own.

There are two popular misconceptions which inhibit experimentation by those operating on a tight budget and time schedule. They are that good food is expensive and requires elaborate preparation. The truth is, it costs far less to put a nutritious, filling family meal on the table than a fast-food, take-away meal. And if you consider the time taken going to pick up a take-away meal, you'd be ahead on that, too.

In order to keep yourself and your child fit and healthy, main meals, snacks and school lunches should be drawn from the five following food groups:

- The high protein group—meat, fish, eggs, dried beans, peas, nuts.
- The cereal group—wholemeal bread, rice, whole grain cereals.
- The high calcium group—milk and cheese.
- Fruits and vegetables.
- Fats and oils—found in butter, margarine and vegetable oils.

Ideally, you should eat something from each food group every day. This may require you to change your shopping habits and restock your food cupboard and refrigerator. But once the changeover is made, you will have learned to do without junk food—high sugar biscuits, cakes, high salt chips, artificially flavoured, artificially coloured, deep fried corn puffs, lollies and chocolate—and you will find you are actually spending less on food than you were before. As a basis for comparison, the following two main course recipes are more nutritious and cost less in terms of cash and preparation time than most popular take-away meals.

Chilli con carne

1 clove garlic or garlic salt, 1 small onion (optional)
1 tablespoon polyunsaturated oil
500 gram lean minced beef
1 × 300 gram can of whole kernel corn
1 × 410 gram can of peeled tomatoes (or 4 fresh)
1 × 300 gram can of kidney beans (or equivalent dried beans, soaked overnight)
½–1 teaspoon chilli powder according to taste
half cup stock and gravy thickening powder (optional)

Heat oil in large, flat pan and *sauté* garlic, add meat and turn frequently until lightly browned and crumbly, stir in the rest of the ingredients adding chilli powder last, gradually, to taste, simmer for 20 minutes. Serve with boiled rice (about one cup, dry). Feeds four.

Quiche Lorraine

Sufficient short crust pastry (home made or frozen) to line a 20 cm flan dish
3 eggs
3 rashers of lean bacon (or 3 heaped tablespoons bacon pieces) diced finely
3 tablespoons grated parmesan cheese
1 cup milk
1 dessertspoon dried chives or dried onion flakes
salt, pepper and nutmeg to taste.

Beat eggs and milk until creamy, add parmesan cheese, dried chives or onions, salt and pepper and pour into pastry shell containing chopped bacon; sprinkle with nutmeg and cook in a slow oven (about 150°C) until firm: 45–60 minutes. Serve hot or cold with a mixed salad. Feeds four.

The following suggestions offer nourishing and inexpensive alternatives to tuck-shop or milk-bar lunches for your child, and no lunch at all for yourself:

- Wholegrain bread, cream cheese and raisin sandwiches, carrot sticks wrapped in foil, dried apricots wrapped in foil.
- Wholegrain bread, sliced hardboiled egg and finely sliced celery sandwiches, a tomato, halved, wrapped separately in foil, a mandarin or apple.
- Wholegrain bread, peanut butter and sliced banana sandwiches, dates wrapped separately in foil, an apple.
- Wholegrain bread, Vegemite and sliced cheese sandwiches, carrot sticks in foil, a banana.

Warning

Anorexia nervosa—self induced starvation—more commonly known as the dieting disease, is becoming prevalent among adolescent girls throughout the western world. Nutritional experts believe it is caused by a general unwillingness to grow up and encounter adult problems or by some psychological trauma during puberty.

There is a gradual weight loss at first, which is possibly desirable, depending on the adolescent girl's weight when dieting begins, therefore it is easy to overlook the onset of the disease. But there are symptoms which you can and should watch for if you have an adolescent daughter who is skipping meals or following any self devised diet.

They include:

- Continual rejection of food;
- Hyperactivity—continual exercise, pacing, excessive studying, a frenetic desire to burn up energy;
- Constipation—to the point when she relies, regularly, on laxatives;
- Amenorrhea—irregular or cessation of menstrual periods;
- Vomiting—almost always self induced, this is an important clue to the victim's condition as it indicates unwillingness to digest food even though she may be paying lip service to eating;
- Excessive weight loss, beyond the point of reasonable weight reduction.

6

Your role as custodian parent

Rarely, except in the most amicable circumstances, does a couple on the point of separation and divorce sit down and discuss their future roles as custodian and access parents, in their own interests or those of their child. All too often, the two most important people in the child's life become polarised by their emotional reactions, leaving him in the vacuum they have created, his needs and his wants overlooked completely, or worse, manipulated to punish or reward his parents by one or both of them.

Even if parents do start out with good intentions towards their child, once the legal wheels are set in motion, a subtle change of character can occur, and normally decent, rational men and women who have never before considered blackmail or extortion and would be appalled at the prospect of child abuse, begin to practise all three, with their own child as their unwitting tool and victim.

Counsellors who work with single parent families agree that hostility and anxiety are the two most prevalent and potentially damaging emotional reactions harboured by custodian parents after a marriage breaks down, as they affect both the custodian parent-child relationship and the child's own emotional development.

If these two perfectly understandable reactions to the separation-divorce trauma are not contained and put in their proper perspective by channelling them out to the appropriate people in your support structure (see Chapter Three), you run the risk of hurting the very person you are trying so hard to protect—your child. How does this happen? Let us examine the build-up and the consequences.

By far the most common form of abuse suffered by children during the post separation-divorce period, is the custody-access tug of war, a sinister 'game' played by parents, with assistance from legal advisers and sometimes even court officials.

Psychiatrists and psychologists sifting through the problems of the child victims of this sort of treatment tell of custodian parents deliberately manipulating access rulings to reward or pay back access parents for higher or lower maintenance payments, doling out their children's time in proportion to their former partner's co-operation. And of access parents holding their own children hostage until 'ransom' agreements are made.

Given these circumstances, it is hardly surprising that hostility is one of the overriding factors influencing the relationship between most custodian and access parents in the post separation period, and during the often long and drawn out litigation preceding divorce. If it is allowed to dictate your behaviour towards each other, parental hostility can do your child more lasting harm than the divorce itself.

One of the inescapable responsibilities of parenting is that children model their own attitudes and behaviour on the pattern set for them by their mothers and fathers. If the predominant attitudes your child picks up between you and his other parent are based on anger, resentment and aggression, you may well be establishing this pattern for his own attitudes towards his peers and the people *he* loves for the rest of his life.

As your child's only live-in parent, you are the most constant example he has to follow, so you bear the bulk of the burden of shaping his behaviour, as he has no other parent on hand to use as a basis for comparison. The following case history may give you some idea of the impact of your own attitude towards your former partner (however justified it might be) on your child, and how it could affect his future behaviour.

When Alex left Anna, he took the family savings, what was left in the family cheque account, and the family car. He also took the boat, outboard motor and trailer he had bought with a personal loan secured with Anna as co-signatory. Anna and their children, Emma and Paul, were left with the house (for the time being), its contents, and $14 left over from the previous week's housekeeping money.

If Alex had told Anna he was going, she might have been better able to control her emotional reaction in front of the children later on. But it wasn't until he was located by the police after Anna reported him missing, that she learned he was living with someone else and her marriage was over. When he later forced the sale of their family home to effect a settlement, she resolved to put him out of her life forever.

For a while, she was able to do that because Alex kept his distance, but eventually he wanted to see his children and arrived, one day, to avail himself of an access ruling which entitled him to spend that afternoon with them. It was too much for Anna, who reacted accordingly.

All the bitterness, frustration and anger erupted and spilled out over Alex—and over Emma and Paul, who had run, spontaneously, into their father's arms. Pulling them away from him, Anna shouted and sobbed recriminations and abuse. Although she had to let them go with him, she refused to allow him to set foot in her house for subsequent pick-ups, and made the children wait at the end of the drive when Alex was due to take them out. She also refused to allow Emma and Paul to talk about their father in front of her, and offered them no information about him herself, even to the extent of withholding the date of their next, scheduled access visit.

Within a few weeks, teachers at the children's school noticed a marked deterioration in Emma's previously high standard of work, and serious behavioural problems with Paul, particularly in relation to the male members of the staff. The school principal, unaware of the family's single parent status, sent a note home with Emma, inviting both parents to make an appointment to discuss their children's problems.

When Anna arrived alone and explained the situation, the school principal was able to guess at the root cause of Emma's and Paul's problems from their mother's attitude towards the marriage breakdown and her former husband. Tentatively, she suggested an appointment with the school psychologist.

After several sessions with Emma and Paul, and subsequently, Anna, the psychologist was able to help her to understand that her hostile attitude towards Alex had set a pattern for her children which they were unable to follow, because they still loved their father. The result, for Paul, was that he felt he had to hate *someone* because that was the only acceptable interpretation of the message he was receiving from the person whose love and approval he needed. Unable to hate his father, he turned on his male teachers in the only way a seven year-old knows how: he played up and was rude and disruptive in class.

Emma, on the other hand, had simply given up. She couldn't please her mother if she loved her father; she couldn't please her father if she didn't. And in her small world in which achievement was measured in terms of parental love and approbation, she came to accept the fact that she was a non-achiever, an attitude which flowed on to her school work.

Research among custodian parents indicates a high level of anxiety from the moment a marriage breaks down, based in most cases, on the very real fear of not being able to provide the basic necessities of life for their children (let alone maintain the pre-marriage breakdown standard of living), on a substantially reduced, single parent income.

It is one of the supreme ironies of human nature that, in times of stress, we tend to turn on those we love, instead of *to* them. One of the most tragic side effects of separation and divorce which illustrates this human failing best, is the increased risk of stress-induced physical violence in the parent-child relationship.

A young mother, six months pregnant and left alone with her two-year-old daughter when her husband moved out, tells a moving story of how her fear of the future, in particular her anxiety about being able to provide for her daughter and the new baby she was expecting, drove her to endanger one of the children she was worrying about protecting . . .

'It all happened so suddenly, I didn't have time to set myself up, independently, before Stan left. I wasn't even aware that he was unhappily married. He didn't have anyone else, he just came home one night, told me he couldn't take the responsibility any more, packed his port and went out.

'We weren't buying the place we lived in, so there was no equity or anything like that to look forward to when we moved out. I borrowed some money off my mother, to pay the next month's rent but she couldn't afford to support me indefinitely, and in my condition, who'd employ me? I really was in a fix. I literally didn't know what would become of us—especially when the baby came. I couldn't eat and I couldn't sleep. I didn't want to take any pills to calm me down because of the baby, and I'm afraid I started over-reacting when Debby needed attention, or cried.

'All I wanted was to be left alone to try to work out how we could live. I knew there were certain authorities I could get in touch with about emergency grants and single parent pensions, but I was afraid they'd take one look at me and say I wasn't capable of looking after Debby so I tried to sort things out myself.

'One night, Debby wouldn't go to sleep. She kept climbing out of her cot and coming into the kitchen and pulling at me, trying to get up onto my lap. My back ached and my head ached from trying to figure out what I'd get if I sold everything we had and moved in with mum for a while, just until I had the baby, and before I really realised what I was doing, I'd picked Debby up and thrown her across the room. She landed against the couch and hit her head on the wooden arm. I remember being surprised to see her there, as if someone else had done this terrible thing to her. And then I saw the blood and that she wasn't moving.

'Fortunately, my mum walked in at that moment and she took Debby and me to the doctor who arranged for me to go into hospital and have a rest until the baby was born, while mum looked after Debby. The social worker at the hospital helped me fill out all the forms and stuff to get the single parent pension, and by the time I had the baby, I had a whole new outlook on life. I wasn't scared any more. I knew it wouldn't be easy, but I also knew there were plenty of people willing to help me if I looked for them. But I still have awful times thinking about what I did to Debby, how close I came to really hurting her, which is why I've joined a parent group which gives you support when you need it, and helps by discussing the difficult side of raising kids . . . '

Sometimes, even the basic tenets of custodian parenthood can become an emotional health hazard for your child if the reaction which triggers them is too intense.

'Smother love'—the result of a combination of overcare, overprotection and overcompensation—can stifle your relationship with your child and stunt his development as a self sufficient, independent human being. It can rob him of his self reliance and turn him into an introspective schemer, setting one parent against the other (or the custodian parent against any other adult who may compete for the child's or his mother's affections) for is own personal gain.

It is perfectly natural for you to want to shield your child from further hurt—from yourself, his other parent or anyone else who may appear to be making life difficult for him. But you must allow him to take a few knocks and disappointments, in and outside the home, if he is to learn to be able to cope with the problems of personal relationships later in life.

Letting little Billy dive into the cookie jar every time he wants a biscuit might make him happy for the moment, but in the long term it can only make him fat (something he may well blame you for when he is an obese adult!). Buying him the biggest and best bike on the street will not make up for the fact his father is not around to help him learn to ride it. And giving him more pocket money than the rest of the kids in the neighbourhood will not win him friends, for envy rarely fosters worthwhile friendships.

By the same token, your child cannot compensate for your lost husband. He cannot share your hopes and dreams for the future, or be expected to provide emotional support for you when things go wrong or life lets you down. If you demand too much of your child's attention, you may end up losing him for good when he is old enough to escape your cloying clutches.

If you really want to do the right thing by your child in your new role as custodian parent, there are several positive aspects of single parenting to concentrate on:

- Make a determined effort to establish a new relationship with your former partner, based on the needs and requirements of your child. You can begin by making regular contact, either by telephone, letter, or if you cannot risk the consequences of personal contact, via a third person, to exchange news of your child's developing skills and problems at home and at school.

- Encourage, but never force, your child to talk about his other parent, his hopes for and his fears about their future relationship. Allow them to communicate regularly by phone and letter between access visits. This will let your child see it's okay to love his other parent, and by lessening his anxiety, could put your own relationship with him on a sounder basis.
- Help your child develop a sense of independence from both parents by guiding him towards an outside interest—a play group if he is a pre-schooler, a gym club or music lessons if he is at primary school, travel and field studies if he's older.
- Develop independent interests of your own which take the pressure off your relationship with your child. An art group, a tennis lesson, charity work, a school support group or a part time job can relieve the more monotonous side of parenting, and put into perspective the drama of whether or not Donnie eats his greens or Melissa wears pink socks with her red skirt.

A final word of advice: don't make a crusade out of parenting. You are not your child's *only* parent; your former partner has responsibilities here too. Encourage him to share school visits, dental checks, cub-scout-guide-calisthenics pick-up and delivery car pools. One day your child will grow up and out of the life support structure you have built for him. If that is *all* you've done with your life, you could find you have nothing left to lean on yourself.

A custodian father faces an extra problem to those just examined for custodian mothers, in that he may feel he has to make a role change involving a whole new way of life if he was previously the family's primary breadwinner.

With his child's mother gone, he may feel he is the obvious person to take over the day to day life support system she provided, shopping for and preparing meals, washing, ironing and mending clothes, and the thousand and one similar, repetitive chores that make up the care structure a child—and a husband—usually takes for granted. On the other hand, he recognises the need to keep on working at his regular job in order to furnish the money to maintain the standard of living he has set for his family.

If you are a custodian father contemplating full time parenting on a single parent pension, you may be well advised to try to arrange an extended period of leave from your place of employment as a trial period for your proposed role switch, to see how both you and your child(ren) cope.

Family therapists have found that the unaccustomed pressures on housebound men, particularly those new to the situation, with infants or pre-school aged children to care for can reduce the strongest man to his emotional breaking point if he is not prepared for the change in his lifestyle. You may well be able to change nappies, prepare nourishing meals or send your child to school immaculately turned out, but the loneliness of your long-term, single, shut-in status which, in most cases, is such a change from your previous work force pace, may be too much for you to bear.

If you can take a month or two off work to get your bearings, you should be able to work out a routine, together with key people from your support structure (see Chapter Three) to take over the surrogate mother role on a trial basis. And if you find it doesn't work for you, you can use the rest of your leave to interview housekeepers, or organise relatives to care for your child when you revert to your more familiar father role.

7

Your role as access parent

Just as a custodian parent's hostility towards an access parent can rub off on their child, so too can the hostility an access parent often feels towards the child's custodian parent.

No matter how much each parent may love their child, or how earnestly they want to preserve his happiness, unless a couple on the point of separating can sit down and discuss their continuing relationship with each other as it affects their child, they will almost certainly inflict some degree of emotional abuse on him, directly or indirectly, as a by-product of their reactions to each other's behaviour.

Access parents questioned about the causes of their hostility towards custodian parents put resentment and fear at the top of the list. The resentment usually stems from the rejection an access parent experiences when he moves out of the family home (or his wife leaves, taking their child with her). Regardless of who caused the marriage breakdown, the sympathy and attention of relatives, friends and welfare workers is focused on the custodian parent and her problems. And suddenly, from being titular head of the family, he is reduced to the status of an outsider, *persona non grata* in his own home, his rights and responsibilities dictated to him by strangers, his income apportioned by some remote authority for the next five, ten, even eighteen years.

The fear an access parent experiences is a very basic one—surprising in its intensity to even the most irresponsible, non-paternal access parent: that he may lose or be lost by his child for ever.

The most common reaction to these new-found anxieties is for an access parent to strike back, or out, at his child's custodian parent, the person he considers, rightly or wrongly, to be the cause of them. Counsellors trying to establish a tenable relationship between separated parents in their children's interests, tell of access parents deliberately delaying or withholding maintenance payments in order to 'get even with' custodian parents, or make them agree to regular, lesser amounts than the court may have stipulated. Some extend access visits by hours or even days, or 'snatch' their children from school for unscheduled visits in retaliation for what they feel are unfair custody-access rulings. Only rarely are the children the intended victims of this sort of emotional warfare, but they are inevitably the *real* victims.

With this in mind, one of the first responsibilities of your new access parent role should be to recognise your hostility towards your child's other parent for what it is—a natural reaction—then put it out of your mind so that you can work at building a new relationship with your former partner which will give your child the emotional security he deserves.

This may not be easy, at first, as both of you will probably be on the defensive, especially if you parted on anything less than amicable terms with all the problems of custody and access, maintenance and financial settlements sorted out satisfactorily prior to the walk out. It is not unusual for parents caught in the early stages of the separation-divorce trauma to find it impossible to communicate rationally about anything—even the welfare of their child which is probably the only thing they have left in common.

If you feel that there is any risk of a row erupting in front of your child whom you try for personal contact with your former partner, you are more likely to establish some sort of *détente* through a third person. A mutual friend you both respect could act as go-between, or maybe a relative that the custodian parent trusts to have your child's interests at heart. (Legal representatives are fine for sealing any agreement you may subsequently reach, but, as a rule, they are regarded with suspicion by both sides during early negotiations.) If there is really no one you know or trust well enough to intercede on your behalf, you might consider writing to your former partner. When you do, try to avoid the 'you made me' approach. State your requests and suggestions clearly and courteously, and give her time to consider them—especially if you have had only limited interest in your child's welfare up to this point.

Another avenue of continuing involvement with your child may be through his school. You still have the right to show interest in his education, and if your former partner refuses to keep you informed of his progress, you should approach the school principal for information and direction.

Men and women who reach higher levels of responsibility in our education system are usually fairly shrewd judges of character and intent, and if you are genuinely interested in your child's academic and emotional development, you should find not only the principal but all his teachers sympathetic and co-operative. You could even attend some of the school functions and parent-teacher meetings without risking a confrontation with your child's other parent, by requesting a clearance from your former partner or the school principal.

You could also request copies of school notices and end of term reports to support your efforts to maintain your involvement. If your former partner will not co-operate by supplying them, your child's school principal probably will. This is even more likely if your child is having trouble adjusting to his new, single parent status, which may show up as erratic behaviour, or a drop in his achievement level.

The value of an access parent's continued involvement in a child's school life—provided it doesn't result in embarrassing scenes—is often overlooked by both parents, even in the most amicable of marriage breakdowns. The following case history may serve to show you just how important you are to your child and his school life . . .

Amanda was seven when she first experienced stomach pains. It was during an art class at the primary school she attended, and after ascertaining that the child had had nothing upsetting to eat during the preceding few hours, Amanda's teacher took her along to the sick room for a short lie down.

By the time the art class had finished, Amanda had recovered. She didn't seem to mind missing out on the card making session the rest of the class had enjoyed, and went on to take part in the physical education period which followed with no apparent ill effects. That was in September. By the end of the third term, with Christmas approaching rapidly, Amanda's stomach aches returned with increasing frequency, and her mother was notified when they appeared to become more intense.

Amanda's family doctor examined the child but could find no apparent cause of her discomfort. He questioned her mother about her diet and learned nothing which threw any light on the little girl's problem. It wasn't until Amanda's teacher was clearing out her pupils' chair bags that she came across a number of screwed up pieces of paper, all with incomplete drawings and half finished greetings on them, which gave her—and the rest of those concerned about Amanda's mystery stomach illness—a clue to the cause of the problem.

Gently, she questioned the child about the greeting cards—each one of several attempts to produce a father's day card and a Christmas card for 'mum and dad'. Tearfully, Amanda explained she hadn't been able to finish her cards because she didn't have a daddy at home to give them to. The stomach aches were simply her way of expressing her inability to complete the project.

With Amanda's mother's permission, the school principal wrote to the child's father, inviting him to come to the school to discuss his daughter's dilemma and view her work. With Amanda proudly holding his hand her father visited the art room to look at all the cards the children had prepared for their parents that Christmas. After that, Amanda's stomach aches disappeared . . . and her father made sure he attended at least one school function a term.

In certain situations, because an access parent has moved away from the city or state in which his children live, it may not be possible to continue to provide the support they need in person. And the role of access parent becomes a more difficult one, and could break down completely.

If you have moved away from your former family, or your child's other parent has taken him to live too far away for you to visit him, or for him to visit you frequently, there are other means of maintaining the continuity of your father role which family therapists agree is vital to him at any age. You could, for instance, instigate a writing relationship. Even a pre-schooler can appreciate a picture postcard with 'I LOVE YOU' printed on the back over the name 'DADDY', if you can persuade someone to read it to him.

The basis for a continuing relationship is trust, so if you plan to start writing to your child, you must be prepared to write regularly or you could subject him to days or even weeks of suspense, wondering if you haven't written because he wrote something to upset you, or worse, you have simply forgotten him.

A letter of his own can provide your child with a valuable public and private crutch on which to lean in times of stress and self doubt related to his single parent status, or even something quite outside the sphere of your separation and divorce (children do have other problems!). His crisis can be a temporary one—his mother won't let him have a pony for Christmas—or a more enduring drama. Either way, the evidence, held in his hand (or kept under his pillow), that he has someone of his own to confide in, discuss the problem with, or who simply cares enough to post a letter, acts as a safety valve for otherwise pent up emotions. He might never reach the point of actually writing down his troubles and mailing them to you, but your letter lets him know the lines of communication are open if he wants to.

Communication is what the access parent-child relationship is really all about from now on. The amount of communication between you will determine your status as a part time or full time parent whether you see your child every day, every week, every month, or only now and then.

Because you are the adult and, in your child's eyes, leader of your two man team, it is up to you to take the initiative setting up the lines of communication. You might try regular phone calls (but not just before bed time or when he's in bed), a flow of post cards from anywhere you happen to go, or you could draw pictures for each other, or exchange items of interest from newspapers or magazines depending on your child's age, interests and abilities.

If you have had little or no communication with your child (for whatever reason) and would like to re-establish contact, you would be wise to try a circuitous route rather than surprise your son or daughter with a direct approach.

If you can rely on the co-operation of his other parent, make contact with her first, explaining what you have in mind and perhaps enclosing an unsealed note to your child. (By leaving the note unsealed you relieve your former partner of any anxiety she may have regarding your intentions.) Follow this up with a phone call, and if you feel the time is right, speak with your child. If there has been any lengthy gap in your relationship, it's a good idea to keep it light at first, without undue emotion, until both you and your child (and his other parent) have established the basis for a deeper, on-going relationship.

Whatever means of communication you decide on to maintain your permanent parent status after you move out of the family home, there is one golden rule you must keep if you want to preserve the trust you have built up between yourself and your child: never abuse it by using it to find out about your former partner.

Encourage him to talk freely about his own hopes, fears, worries and doubts, but don't question your child about his mother's life, where she goes, what she does or with whom she does it. Children have an uncanny sixth sense and know when they are being put on the spot. The anxiety that fear of disloyalty—to either parent—can cause a child can have serious and lasting emotional consequences. If he is worried or concerned about his mother, or some aspect of her life as it relates to him, the chances are good, if you've gained his confidence, that he'll tell you anyway.

One of the best ways to supplement access periods and spend more time with your child than the court has decreed (providing your former partner agrees, of course), is to offer to continue to chauffeur your child to one or some of his after-school activities. While the time you actually spend with him may be brief, you can give—and receive—a great deal in the way of support and reassurance on a short car trip to cubs, brownies, calisthenics or swimming. But before you commit yourself to the once-a-week responsibility, you must be prepared to keep it up. Although it may seem improbable to an access parent desperate to maintain a full time parent role after an access ruling you may consider to be loaded against you, there is a danger, in the initial, emotional stages of separation from your child, of letting him down if you find you cannot maintain the standards you have set yourself.

Therapists working with children suffering the classic symptoms of rejection in their early teens, tell a repetitious story of missed access visits, dwindling correspondence, infrequent phone calls and forgotten birthdays. It is far better for your child to have less contact with you on a regular basis than sporadic bursts of frequent visits, letters or telephone calls followed by periods of apparent indifference or neglect.

If you need further evidence of the importance of sustained fathering—even long distance and well spaced—consider the story of a girl we shall call Cathy, who tells how the father she had not seen for nearly thirteen years, provided the support she needed in a personal crisis when those who had been around her all her life could not.

'I was three when my mum and dad split up . . . I never really knew why, but I got the impression from my mum that dad was a bit of a louse, although she never said exactly why.

'Anyway, I had what I guess you'd call a fairly ordinary upbringing . . . my mum married again and had another couple of kids and I felt their dad was really my dad, too until I was about fifteen, I'd say it was. That was when I sort of blossomed out, as he put it.

'I started going out with boys, nowhere special because none of the boys I knew had any money—just hanging around the milk bar down the road, going to the youth club, that sort of thing. Some nights I'd stay out late, I'll admit that—say, until 11 or 12 at night, of a Saturday—and one night, I didn't get home until after one.

'Boy, was there trouble when I got in! Mum and dad were both up, looking like World War Three had begun and they both started yelling at me as I walked in the door. They didn't give me a chance to say where I'd been, or what I'd been doing. In fact, a friend of mine had fallen off his motorbike and a few of us had gone to the hospital with him and waited in the casualty department until he was admitted.

'In any case, it suddenly didn't matter any more. It was obvious what they thought of me, mum even came out with it . . . "you're just like your father", she said, meaning my real father, not the one I called dad.

'Okay, I said, if that's what you think I'll clear out. I don't think I really meant it at the time, but they weren't giving me any chances to take it back.

'The following morning, mum told me to pack my bag and she'd take me over to gran's for a few weeks, until she'd had time to think what she was going to do with me. Maybe she didn't really mean what she was saying, either, at the time . . . I can see how I must have driven her to it, to a degree, staying out and acting up and all that. But still, when your mother tells you you're not wanted, it finishes something. I don't really know how to put it, but I knew I could never go back home and feel I really belonged, ever again.

'Just as we drove up to gran's place, she handed me this envelope. She said she'd been keeping it for me until I needed it. It wasn't until after she'd left, and I was having a cup of tea with gran, that I opened it. Inside I found a bank book, a savings account in my name, with regular amounts deposited twice a year, on my birthday and Christmas, for the past thirteen years by my real father.

'I can't tell you what that did for me. It wasn't the money because that didn't amount to all that much, really. It was knowing that I had someone else of my own to turn to. Someone who had cared enough about me all those years to remember my birthday and Christmas without me having to appreciate it, without anyone ever knowing.

'I live with my father now and I've learned why he kept in

the background for so long. He admits he caused the break-up by playing around a bit, which mum couldn't take, and when she married again, he thought we'd all have a better chance of being a proper family, which was what mum had always wanted, if he kept out of the way. I've patched things up with mum and dad, but my father and I accept each other just as we are, no questions asked, it's a very special feeling . . . '

8

Taking the stress out of access visits

- Children as young as two and three years left waiting on the footpath by custodian parents for access parents who may or may not show up . . .
- Infants pulled screaming from custodian parents' arms and forcibly restrained in access parents' cars . . .
- Five and six year olds deliberately unsettled by custodian parents, prior to access visits, so that they are 'unwell' when access parents arrive to take them out . . .
- Seven and eight year olds kept out until midnight, returning home fatigued and distressed, not knowing which parent to cling to for comfort and rest . . .
- Children of all ages dumped at the end of their driveways by mutual agreement of both parents to avoid personal contact, left to cross the no-man's land between their mothers and fathers, alone . . .
- Parents physically fighting while their children try to pull them apart, before or after access visits . . .
- Children deliberately over-fed and over-indulged by access parents, in order to make the immediate post-access period unhappy and uncomfortable in custodian parents' homes . . .
- Children arriving for, and from, access visits bruised and weeping . . .

- Nine and ten year-olds reverting to bed-wetting after access visits . . .
- Brothers and sisters separated according to access parents' preferences, the rejected child left at home with or without warning . . .
- Children from two to twelve years under regular psychiatric care to help them cope with access visits and the constant change of environment and parental control . . .
- Symptoms of psychosomatic illness including asthma, bronchitis, vomiting and diarrhoea, and total rejection of both parents, sometimes combined with outbursts of physical violence, before and after access visits . . .

These are just some of the stories told by parents, grand parents and other relatives, and in some cases the children themselves, seeking advice on how to cope with one of the most difficult aspects of separation and divorce—access visits.

It was always the intention of the *Family Law Act* to provide the best possible opportunity for both parents to continue to have a meaningful, on-going relationship with their child/ren after divorce. Consequently, with 'quality time' seen to be at a premium on weekends, most access orders were made for children to spend alternate weekends with their custodial and access parents. This was fine in theory and, indeed, worked well for children of parents who had separated on amicable terms, or were able to temper any residual hostility with the need to comply with the spirit as well as the letter of such orders.

But it soon became evident that for children caught in the middle of their parents' unresolved conflict, the constant shuttling to and fro between hostile, point-scoring parents carried a significant risk of emotional and even physical abuse. This was particularly evident in the case of infants and very young children.

With the availability of more Family Court counsellors, the growth of community-based counselling services, and the introduction of legal representation of children involved in cases argued in the Family Court, emphasis has been placed, in recent years, on mediation prior to cases being heard in court. There has also been a developing awareness of the need for flexibility in access orders, to better meet the changing needs of children—and their parents. Consequently, the number of disputed custody and access hearings that come before the court has, thankfully, fallen in recent years.

Nevertheless, given the vagaries of human behaviour and the influence of external pressures, even the most carefully conceived conditions for custody and access can fail. If you believe your child may be at risk emotionally or physically during time spent with your ex-partner, you should immediately seek help from your family doctor, your lawyer and/or a Family Court counsellor.

If you believe an offence has been committed against your child, you should not hesitate to contact the police. In cases of suspected sexual abuse, the Family Court can, mindful of its duty to protect the interests of your child, suspend access without having positive proof that an offence has occurred. The court will then make the relevant orders to ensure the proper investigations are carried out and duly processed.

For parents facing the prospect of implementing custody or access orders now, or in the future, here are a few simple guidelines to help facilitate a smooth transition to a positive new relationship for all concerned.

What a custodian parent can do

However much you may resent your former partner for his previous attitude or behaviour, if you have any concern for the emotional stability of your child, you must resolve to make the time he spends with his other parent as pleasant as possible.

How pleasant it is depends on you as much as his other parent, because the signals he receives from you about the forthcoming visit will influence his own attitude towards it almost as much as if you sat him down and told him whether or not to enjoy it.

Depending on your child's age and ability to comprehend, you should begin the 'warm up' to the proposed access visit well in advance of the due date . . . say, two or three days for infants or primary school children, longer for older children. Encourage your child to put aside projects to share with his other parent; jig-saw puzzles, a toy which needs mending, even school work are all fine because they invite involvement.

Try to remember the good things about your marriage and talk about them with your child. Offer as much information as you can (without prejudice) about what your former partner is doing now, where he is living, with whom your child is likely to come into contact. Psychiatrists have found the things which worry children on the access shuttle most are: what sort of house they will be staying in, what size bed they will sleep in, whether or not they will be allowed to take their favourite toys, if there is a telephone in the house (just knowing you are within reach by telephone is reassuring even if the visit does not involve an overnight stay), if there is a garden to play in, how many—if any—children will be around with whom they can play.

Clothes play an important part in how a child feels and reacts to any given situation. Avoid giving into the temptation to show your former partner (and his girl-friend/new wife) how well you look after your child by dressing him in his best for the visit. Best clothes give a sense of occasion when the aim of the exercise is to allow the access parent and child to maintain a degree of normality in their relationship. Children are invariably more relaxed in play clothes, so set aside the sort of outfit your child would wear around his own home for the access period, unless specifically requested to include something more dressy. It is also a good idea to lay out an extra set of clothes, even if your child is only going out for the afternoon—accidents happen and wet pants or a coke-splashed dress can make an otherwise happy day miserable.

Invite your child to discuss the upcoming access visit with you. Find out if he is worried about anything or any aspect of the time he will be spending with his other parent. Many small children are acutely embarrassed about wetting the bed, for instance, and need to be reassured that their fathers are able to carry out the recovery operation. (One seven year old refused to get into bed at her access parent's house because she discovered there was no rubber sheet between the mattress and the underblanket, and she was afraid she would get into trouble if she wet through to the mattress of the pretty new bed her father had bought for her.)

If you discover something is worrying your child about the visit, communicate his fears by telephone or letter to his other parent so that he can help put your child's mind at rest when he is with him.

You can take the tension out of your own attitude towards access visits by programming something for yourself for the time your child is with his other parent. Some hobby you've always wanted to try, a visit to a gallery, a movie or a show, lunch out with friends, followed by an afternoon of window shopping—anything rather than sitting at home, wondering what is going on in your ex-partner's home.

If you are at all worried about your own or your former partner's reaction to personal confrontation at hand-over time, arrange for a third party to be present with you, or instead of you, when your former partner calls. If you really cannot tolerate the thought of him coming into your home, you might arrange to have your child picked up and dropped off at his grandparents' house or some other place he enjoys visiting.

It is quite common for children of newly separated or divorced parents to become over dependent on, and physically cling to, the custodian parent for some time after the break-up. This is especially so with infants and younger primary school-aged children who fear that having lost one parent, they may well lose the other if they let her out of their sight. Tears flow at the prospect of even the shortest separation, and in some cases a child's distress level can reach hysteria if it is not handled correctly. Unfortunately, access pick ups often spark this sort of reaction in children which, in turn, triggers the very opposite behaviour to that required of the parents. Instead of remaining calm and supportive of each other as well as their child, they tend to turn on each other which upsets their child even more.

If your child is at all 'clingy' or becomes upset when you are out of sight, you could do a lot to defuse the hand over situation if you take it in stages. For instance, you might include it in a visit to gran's, taking him there 'to meet daddy' . . . or you might take him to daddy's place and once he's settled, take your leave.

But never, never leave without telling your child you are going—the sudden realisation that you are missing can be devastating to a small child who depends on you for his very existence. Always tell your child when you will return for him, or when he will be brought back to you (littlies have a hard time measuring time spans, but relating time to meals helps and 'one sleep and wake up' explains an overnight). Therapists have found that leaving something of yours with your child to 'mind' for you while you are apart offers reassurance that you will come back for him.

In your child's interests, as much as those of his other parent, make sure you communicate regularly, by telephone or letter, with your former partner to keep him informed of your child's developing skills, likes or dislikes, and any difficulties he may be having with his behaviour or school work and, most important, his state of health.

When the all important day arrives for his other parent to pick him up, give your child the best possible start to it by your own attitude. The hours ahead may be difficult enough for him to cope with, without having to worry about you crying alone, at home, or being angry and resentful when he returns.

When the visit is over and your child comes home, take him down gradually off the 'high' the excitement will probably have caused. It is not unusual for children returning from an access visit to be loud, rude, aggressive or tearful—all symptoms of emotional upset or over excitement in children of all age groups. And above all, don't question your child about his other parent . . . if he is sure of your love and support, he'll probably tell you everything that happened while he was away from you, anyway.

What an access parent can do

One of the most difficult aspects of access visits, as far as access parents are concerned, can be what to do with your child when you've got him! Removed from the familiar environment of the casual encounters the father-child relationship is usually built on—pottering in the garden, driving to school, clearing out the garage, working around the house on a Sunday morning—the exchange between you and your child can become stilted in the synthetic setting of a restaurant, cinema or similar 'special' venue.

By far the best place you can take your child, at least initially, on access visits is your own home. It doesn't matter if it is only a two-roomed flat, you can get closer over a glass of milk and a sandwich at a kitchen table than almost anywhere outside.

If you share a place with others who might invade your privacy with your child, you could arrange to spend time alone with him at his grandparents' home, or some other place in which he feels comfortable. If you do schedule outings, make sure you don't set up a tiring itinerary. The excitement of the visit, plus the build-up will take a lot out of him, and you may find him drooping visibly long before your access period is at its end. Should this happen, you won't lose face with your child or your former partner if you telephone his home and arrange to take him home early.

Whatever his age, avoid questioning your child about his other parent. Children have a strong sense of loyalty and should either parent appear to abuse the other's privacy most children clam up. You could find this may put an end to the rapport you have established and you will miss out on the confidences your child really wants to share.

Don't expect your child to enjoy being with you all the time. If he were home with his other parent, there would probably be periods when he would be bored or tired, his tummy might ache or he'd be wanting his friends. It helps to relieve the pressure on both of you to enjoy the time you spend together, if you make sure you have the materials on hand for him to amuse himself when conversation flags or time hangs heavy. These will, of course, vary with your child's interests, gender and capabilities, but may include jig-saw puzzles, postcards, scrap books, old magazines and a pot of glue, a model battleship or aircraft, some new doll's clothes, building kits or possibly the ingredients for a cooking exercise.

The main purpose of the *Family Law Act* in respect to relaxed access rulings is to help access parents maintain the continuity of parenting as far as it may be possible, bearing in mind the fact they are no longer living with their children. If you are experiencing difficulty maintaining the degree of involvement in your child's life you hope for, there are a number of ways you can play a continuing, if part-time, role in his life.

Keeping yourself informed of his progress at school (see

Chapter Seven) gives you a basis for communication. You can and should talk to (not harass) your child about his school work, perhaps suggesting you help him with a project, his homework or any problem requiring extra attention. You might also arrange with his other parent to pick him up and drop him off after school activities outside your scheduled visits.

Small children enjoy growing things, so if you've space outside, or even a window box, you can share the on-going excitement of planting seeds and watching them grow, from forking over the earth to watering, fertilising and even picking the flowers or fruits when they mature. Story telling, chapter by chapter, visit by visit, is another way to promote a continuing interest with a small child and it gives you both something to share exclusively and look forward to between visits.

But whatever you do—or don't do—with your child during the hours, days or weeks you spend with him, by far the most critical periods will be collecting him from his home and taking him back again.

If you don't exercise great care to set out and abide by a few, basic ground rules, both you and your child's custodian parent can wipe out all the good your access visits do for him. Even if you loathe each other, contain your hostility long enough to maintain some sort of control when you meet. If you really cannot trust yourself to keep cool, take someone else with you to effect the actual handover so that you can kiss your child hello or goodbye, all smiles, in the car. Alternatively, arrange for the pick up or drop off to take place on neutral territory. As previously suggested, the home of your child's grandparents or some other relative or trusted friend with whom he feels at ease will do well.

Last but by no means least important, make sure that you don't over commit yourself to your child in the early stages of separation and divorce, when you are desperately trying to do the right thing by him. The most precious thing you can share with your child from now on is your time. It is of more value to him than the most extravagant gifts, the most memorable outings. It is far better for him to have a few visits a year that he can rely on, than to be promised frequent contact and be let down.

If you feel you may be late for a pick up or have to cancel a visit—for whatever reason—be sure you give your child plenty of notice of any change of plans. No matter how hard you try to get there on time, or how important it is for you to be somewhere else, if you don't show up at the appointed time, your child may interpret your lateness or non arrival as lack of interest, or worse, lack of love.

9

Sex and the single parent

Marriage breakdown is seldom, if ever, caused by a third person, but once a marriage breakdown occurs, a third person can trigger the separation and subsequent divorce. Whether a husband walks out of the family home into the arms of his secretary or leaves to live alone, sooner or later, human nature being what it is, he is probably going to enter another relationship, or a variety of new relationships and may eventually settle into a permanent one with a new partner.

Although she might not believe it possible at first, the same thing goes for the wife left at home (until the property settlement, anyway), with the child(ren). The time will come when she may want to share her life with someone other than her child. Either way, the child as well as the parents will have to make yet another adjustment to their lives. Just as things are beginning to settle down and everyone is learning to accept the new status quo, it's all change again to make room in the new family picture for two more parents—or at least, potential parents.

If you are contemplating, or are already involved in, a new partnership, you may find you need help to cross the minefield of your child's emotional reaction if the partnership—and your relationship with your child—is to survive the transition period. In view of the different pressures on custodian and access parents in respect to their child, we shall consider the subject of sex and the single parent in two parts.

Sex and the custodian parent

Because of the close proximity of the custodian parent and her child, it is almost impossible for even the most discreet parent to keep a new relationship—even a tentative one—under wraps. Children seem to have built-in antennae which pick up signals that pass right by adults. They are particularly sensitive to their mothers' mood changes, and can react to the threat of a challenge to their position of prime importance on a scale of 1–100 in seconds, according to the degree of security they feel themselves, and in the case of children of separated parents, the amount of loyalty they feel for their live-out parents.

The most common reaction experienced by custodian parents on introducing a potential new partner to their children is hostility. This manifests itself in several ways, depending on the age of the children involved. It can be openly aggressive, or covert; some children cover their hostility with indifference to the point of ignoring the new partner completely, others resort to rudeness, name calling and in the case of older children, sometimes physical abuse.

To give you some idea of the sort of resistance you can expect—and how to overcome it—here are two true life romances (supplied by custodian parents who survived the trauma to live—and love—again), with you in the lead role . . .

You have been separated for some months, and a girl friend invites you to dinner at her home where you meet a rather interesting single man, who, although not marriage material, offers much in the way of companionship during the lonely months ahead. You invite him for afternoon tea, the following Sunday.

Sunday dawns, and for the first time in ages you have some personal purpose to your day apart from performing the family life support functions you carry out with monotonous regularity, every other day. You are up with the lark, singing like one, too, sprinkling smiles over your children like early morning sunshine.

You are too happy and preoccupied with cleaning the house and cooking your world-renowned coffee cake to notice that your children are not sending you sunny smiles back. By the time your friend arrives their expressions are anxious, if not hostile, caused, no doubt, by the fact that mother has been acting like a dill all day, and they cannot understand why.

The bell rings and the violins swell to a crescendo as you open the door and let Bill, or Fred, or whomever, in. You exchange meaningful glances above the children's heads (you think), and brush cheeks. As you turn to lead the way into the living room, Bill says 'G'day' to your seven-year-old son who promptly punches him in the stomach. Your nine-year-old daughter, meanwhile, positions herself determinedly between you and the intruder, where she remains for most of his visit.

The afternoon wears on, and becomes more wearing as the minutes ache by. It appears your children must have rehearsed their performance. Their timing is perfect and their combined effect quite devastating. They have never behaved more aggressively, exhibited worse eating habits or given the front and back doors such a beating.

You watch as Bill battles bravely on, biting back reprimands. At six o'clock, you decide he has endured enough. You can almost see him searching his mind for the svelte little number in the black satin dress inside the wild eyed harridan, holding a squirming boy by the back of his neck while scraping coffee cake off her crumpled skirt.

As you see him to the door you realise this is the moment of truth . . . the *dénouement*. Do you:

- Tell him, tearfully, that you guess your children aren't ready to share you yet, and say, 'Goodbye' . . .
- Interpret the look in his eye (probably correctly) as he

glances over your shoulder at your children, and yell, 'And you too, Buster!', as you slam the door in his face . . .

- Smile, and ask him if you could meet outside your home until you get your children on side, and turn your attention to the little monsters, once he has driven away . . . ?

Experts in family counselling agree that the first reaction is a common cop-out for women in the initial recovery stages of separation and divorce, when they are still low on self-confidence and self-esteem. But they stress it is still a cop-out, because sooner or later, you are going to have to come out of your cocoon and face the world—and the relationships—outside your immediate family.

The second reaction might do if you have come to the conclusion that Bill is a bit of a clod anyway. But there are kinder ways to tell him you've made a mistake, and you could inadvertently be giving your children the green light to behave in a similar manner when you introduce a potential partner you'd like to keep around.

But if you care at all about Bill or your future as a normal, sexual, adult female, you have to opt for the third solution to the sort of problems which can occur when you introduce a new partner to your child (or children).

Accept the fact that your child's behaviour, if it is bad when you introduce your new man, is nothing more sinister than a desperate plea for reassurance that you still love him *best* and won't leave him, as daddy may appear to have done, for someone else. If he is old enough to understand about love and companionship on the adult male to adult female level, explain your need and reassure him that while you will always love and need *him*, your new man can bring a bit more love into the family for you both.

Special care should be taken to make sure your child understands that you don't intend to bring your new man into the picture instead of daddy. Even if your child's other parent is an absolute (expletive deleted) in your opinion, he may still be someone special to his child. Once he can be helped to understand that your new man represents no threat to his own position or, as far as he is concerned, his father's, your child will probably relax and actually enjoy having a man around the house who makes mum happy.

If you have older children in your care, you may be faced with a more difficult challenge when you first introduce the idea of mum operating as a woman. The following scenario shows just how difficult this can be and how you might react . . .

You meet a rather stunning, single executive at a tennis club turn who invites you out for dinner. When he arrives to pick you up at your house, you introduce him to your thirteen year old daughter and they exchange perfunctory courtesies. She watches as you drop your handbag and catch the heel of your shoe in your hem as you stoop to pick it up.

After an enjoyable meal, over which you discover you both have a lot in common, your date, whom we shall call Charles, takes you home. You invite him in for a cup of coffee and a few quiet moments together alone. As you walk up to the front door, you realise you may have had more privacy if you'd stayed in the restaurant.

Although it is almost 1 a.m., the TV is on, along with every light in the house, and the living room is littered with soft drink bottles, chip packets, cassettes and CDs. Your daughter is sprawled on the sofa in shortie pyjamas and football socks. 'Hi!', she mumbles through a mouthful of cornflakes.

You take Charles into the kitchen and park him on a stool at the counter. Plugging in the electric kettle, you hope the noise of the hissing element will drown what you know is going to be a confrontation in the living room. The slanging match which follows could be heard a block away and ends with crude references to your age, your choice of partner and your sense of responsibility as a parent. You react by:

- Slapping your daughter's face . . .
- Telling Charles it was all a terrible mistake and that from now on, you'll stick to tennis . . .
- Asking Charles to make the coffee while you sit down, there and then, and set your daughter straight about your needs as well as hers, after which you give her the choice of going to bed or joining you and Charles for a cup of coffee and a quiet chat . . .

The experts predict that you will most likely react emotionally, and depending on whether your paramount emotion is outrage or embarrassment, will opt for either the first or second alternatives. If you care enough about your future, and the healthy emotional development of your daughter, however, (not to mention Charles!) you would be far better off trying number three.

While Charles is looking for the cups and saucers, explain the facts of your life and hers to your daughter. Tell her that you understand the emotional insecurities of adolescence only too well as you have experienced them twice—once as a teenager and again during the period after your marriage breakdown when you had to learn who you were and how to function as an independent adult all over again.

Let her know you need her just as much as she needs you in the single parent set-up. Explain that just as she must explore new relationships outside the special relationship you and she share, so must you if either of you are to be able to have a life of your own. You might both end up in tears but they won't be tears of anger or frustration. And if Charles is still in the kitchen by the time you've mopped up, he can probably offer your daughter the added assurance of acceptance she needs—football socks and all.

The physical aspect of sex as it applies to a custodian parent is more a matter of trust and timing than of words, however young or old your child is when the situation presents itself. The limitations put on a potential partner when he has to take the baby-sitter home and return to the scene of his passion some half an hour after his desire reached its peak, added to the inhibiting effect of having to carry out his seduction *sotto voce* in case he wakes the child(ren), could put a lot of men off. But you can measure your new man's intentions, to a degree, by the way he is willing to persist, despite these handicaps, or his ability to present innovative alternatives.

Whether or not you are willing to risk running a *cinema verité* version of procreation in front of your child is a matter only you can decide, but behavioural experts believe a succession of sexual encounters with different partners offers your child a bewildering example for him to try to copy when he is searching for his own set of values later on.

This is not to say that all physical expressions of love or even mutual attraction should be banned in front of your child. Hugs, kisses, cuddles, pats and special smiles offer healthy evidence of easy sexuality which your child can understand and accept and store for future reference.

Sex and the access parent

The big advantage an access parent has over a custodian parent in exploring new partnerships and their effect upon his child, is that he can develop a relationship to the stage where he has a good idea whether it will work out for him before he tries it out on his child. He also has time to prime his new partner and his child, separately, so that when they do meet, much of the spadework has been done, and their relationship can grow unhindered by uncertainty or insecurity.

Nevertheless, just as a custodian parent and her new partner face the imposing hurdle of her child's loyalty to his or her other parent, so do an access parent and his new partner in reverse. An access parent also faces an additional problem, which, if he is not aware of it or fails to recognise it, can lead to a heartbreaking let-down for his child and put even the strongest new partnership at risk.

Somewhere in the back of the minds of most children of separated and divorced parents, is nurtured the hope that their mother and father will one day be reunited and they can all live happily ever after, together, again. And, in a child's mind, if the access parent is the one who actually left the family home, he is, logically, the one to work on to come back. While reconciliation may be the furthest thing from the parents' minds when they are setting up new partnerships, it is seldom very far from the surface of their child's . . . as you can see from the following case history.

Kirsty was nine when her father and mother split up. She didn't really understand why they decided to go their separate ways—whenever they met, they were friendly, and they talked a lot and sometimes laughed on the phone. Secretly, she felt sure they would get back together again, just like she had seen it happen on the movies and on television. So it came as something of a shock, one Sunday afternoon when her father arrived to take her out, to find another lady sitting in mummy's seat beside him in his car.

Kirsty's fears were allayed, somewhat, by the casual manner in which her father treated the young woman, and the child filed her away in her mind as one of the ladies who worked for daddy at his shop and sometimes went out to measure curtains with him. But when Kirsty's father picked her up the following Saturday, the woman was in the car again.

The warning signals went up and stayed up, fluttering fiercely, when the woman got out of the car at daddy's place and walked into the kitchen and started doing the sort of things mummy always did for Kirsty and her father. Although she wasn't sure what exactly was going on, one thing Kirsty did know—she didn't want another mummy and she didn't want daddy to have another mummy either, so something had to be done to get rid of the other woman.

When her father went to sit next to the woman at the kitchen table, Kirsty pushed past him and sat there instead. When the woman tried to sit near her father on the sofa when they were all watching TV later that afternoon, Kirsty dived between them and snuggled smugly up to her dad. Whenever the lady would try to speak, Kirsty interrupted with a story about something mummy did or said or saw or told her.

At bed time, Kirsty went through her entire repertoire, beginning with calling for drinks of water to rushing down the stairs feigning fear of the dark. By the time she finally fell asleep, her father was thoroughly upset, but strangely, the lady just kept on knitting and smiling.

When she awoke early the next morning, Kirsty padded along to her father's bedroom to apologise for her behaviour the night before. If she could just talk to him by himself, everything would be all right between them, again, and they could telephone mummy and laugh and talk together like they usually did when she stayed at her father's place for the weekend. But as she tiptoed into her father's room, she found someone else in there with him. It was the lady, and they were whispering and laughing together, and Kirsty knew, with awful certainty, that her mother had been replaced. Her father found her sobbing on the back step some time later, her case packed, waiting to go home . . .

Where older children are concerned, loyalty to the custodian parent and resentment of the intrusion of an outsider into what is left of the family circle (which can be interpreted as a desperate wish to hold the family together, despite the separation or divorce) can lead to physical violence between parent and child, or worse, the complete breakdown of the access parent-child relationship.

If you are experimenting with, or are committed to a new partnership, don't dump it in your child's lap as a *fait accompli*—break it to him gently, step by step, explaining your need for the kind of companionship only an adult male to adult female relationship can provide, at the same time reaffirming your need for the companionship and love only he can give you.

Your child will come to terms with your new partnerships much more easily, of course, if both parents offer each other mutual support whenever the subject is brought up. While you may not be able to accept the inevitability of new partnerships in the early stages of separation and divorce, they do play an essential part in your recovery. A new partner usually brings the welcome relief of love and laughter into your life, but most important, hope for a happier future. All of which flows on to your child.

10

Some useful reminders

Give yourself and your child time to progress through the various stages of recovery after you and your partner split up—this could take up to eighteen months or even longer.

- Be prepared for extreme emotional reactions during the recovery period, from yourself, your former partner and your child.
- Don't shut yourself in with your unhappiness. Reach out for help from family and friends and from professional trained community-based counsellors. You can access these through your local community health centre, your religious affiliations and the telephone directory. If your child is at school, set up an independent life-line for him by talking about your changed circumstances with the school counsellor.
- Make the most of support facilities available to you. Contact the relevant authorities in your area for information about the help you are entitled to from federal and state sources. This may include legal aid, cash grants, temporary accommodation, home help and regular allowances.
- Don't leave your child in the dark about what is happening all around him. Fear of the unknown is far more devastating to a child than even the harshest reality. Tell him as much of the truth as he is able to cope with, and answer any questions he may have, simply and honestly as far as

you can. It helps if you can win the co-operation of your former partner when you tell your child about the marriage breakdown.

- Whatever you think about your former partner and his (or her) behaviour prior to and after the marriage breakdown, avoid the temptation to indulge in character assasination when discussing him (her) with your child. Remember, it's his other parent you are talking about. If you challenge his love and loyalty for his other parent, he could end up rejecting you, too, and then he'd have no one to turn to.
- Don't confuse your child by sending out contradictory signals about the situation or your feelings. Make sure what you say tallies with how you say it. For instance, you can only confuse your child and cause him further anxiety if, when he sees you crying and asks what is the matter, you say, 'Nothing'.
- No matter who contributed most to the breakdown of your marriage and the subsequent separation and divorce, don't dwell on guilt or revenge. Put the past behind you and use your energies to concentrate on building a new life for yourself and your child.
- While there is a need to maintain discipline in both the custodian and the access parents' homes, take care not to confuse your child's natural reactions to the new order of things, or an unfamiliar environment with unfounded bad behaviour. Anxiety, insecurity and confusion often manifest themselves as rudeness, aggression and even violence in children of all ages. Find out *why* your child is behaving unacceptably, and then decide what to do about it.
- Emotional upset often results in loss of appetite or the inclination to prepare proper meals. A poor diet can be directly linked with poor health, anti-social behaviour and low achievement levels. Make what you and your child eat

counts. You don't have to eat junk food on a limited income—nutritious food often costs far less.

- If you or your child feel unwell, inform your family doctor about your domestic circumstances, as well as your symptoms. He needs to know about the possible influence of anxiety, stress, and family dynamics to be able to treat you properly.
- Keep in regular contact with your child's teachers and after-school activity leaders, so that you can help him through the rough spots together.
- Try to be a little more available to your child than you might have been before the marriage breakdown. Encourage but never force him to discuss the situation, his hopes and fears for the future, his concern about his relationship with his other parent.
- Don't get into a competitive, over compensating cycle with your former partner. Children find the tension this generates uncomfortable, and some develop the undesirable trait of playing one parent off against the other, for consideration or reward, as a consequence.
- Remember the best parts of your marriage and share them with your child. The past couldn't have been *all* bad and your child needs to grow up with good feelings about his beginnings.
- Don't demand loyalty from your child to the point of excluding his other parent from his thoughts, consideration, life. A child's affections often appear to swing from one parent to the other and this exhibits a normal, healthy balance. If you ask him to choose between you, he may reject you both.
- Do try to build a life of your own, apart from your natural involvement with your child. You can't live your life through or exclusively for him; he cannot replace your hus-

band (wife) as your partner in life. For his sake, as well as your own, you should strive for independent coexistence.

- Even if you know your marriage is dead, that there is absolutely no hope of reconciliation with your former partner, don't expect your child to accept the finality of separation or divorce as soon as you do. Children often nurture a secret hope that their parents will get together again. Their frustration when this fails to happen is a common cause of upset in custodian and access parents' homes.
- Continuing anger or bitterness between his parents will injure your child far more than their separation and divorce. Work on establishing a new relationship with your former partner, with your child's interests and well-being in mind. You don't have to like each other to do this, but you may discover a new, mutual respect when you see the settling effect it has on him.
- Keep your child's other parent informed about his progress at school, include him (her), whenever possible, in school activities and after-school hobbies and interests. Keep him (her) up to date with any new likes and dislikes, difficulties and developing skills. Let him (her) know about any problems with health or behaviour.
- Prepare your child for access visits well in advance of the due date. Set aside some continuing project for him to show or share with his other parent—school work, a jig-saw puzzle, some new toy or interest, a broken doll's crib or a bent bike—anything that will bridge the gap between them, and invite the support your child needs from his access parent.
- Don't dress your child in his best for access visits. Clothes affect the way a child feels, as well as the way he looks. Send him out in the sort of gear he feels most comfortable in, unless requested to provide the appropriate clothes for some special outing.

- Access visits are unsettling enough for children in the initial stages, without them having to endure an exchange of hostilities between parents at handover time. If you anticipate trouble between you and your former partner when you meet, arrange for a third person to be there with or instead of you at the appointed time.
- If you have arranged to pick up your child for an access visit, be punctual to the minute. If you are unavoidably delayed, make sure he gets a message giving him the reason and a new time, *before* he experiences the let down of your non-arrival. Lateness on the part of an access parent is often interpreted by a child as lack of interest—especially if he is the one who walked out on the family (for whatever reason).
- If you have arranged to pick up your child *from* an access visit, be sure you arrive exactly at the appointed time. A small child may wonder whether you will ever come back to pick him up if he is left in a strange environment, and the anxiety he experiences is only increased if you fail to show up when you said you would.
- Just as the custodian parent has a responsibility to keep the access parent informed about their child's anxieties, fears, problems, new skills and so on, the access parent should let the custodian parent know of any problems, upsets or achievements logged at his home during access visits. This sort of feedback is essential if your child is to receive the continuity of support and encouragement he needs for healthy emotional and physical growth.
- Access visits should never be used to check on the other parent. A child should never be pumped for information. He must feel the love he gets from each parent is unconditional and not dependent on giving the right or wrong answers to either one.

- Be prepared for hostility and outrageous behaviour from your child, whatever his age, when you first introduce the idea of potential new partnerships to him. This is an entirely normal, understandable reaction when he feels his own security threatened (he might be replaced in your affections), or his loyalty to his other parent challenged (he might be expected to replace his father/mother with someone else in *his* affections). If he is old enough to understand about adult male-adult female relationships, explain that it makes no difference to your need for the relationship you share with your child, or the one he shares with his other parent. An anxious infant or a small child can be reassured by increased evidence of affection for him (her) when your new partner is around until he realises there is no contest.
- Look for the positive aspects of your future as a single parent. Many people report a power surge from the realisation that they are free to make their own choices and take control of their own lives. This gives them the confidence to reach out for new skills to improve their job options and tap into new interest groups.

A final word . . . help your child through separation and divorce by doing something positive for yourself every day. The benefits will flow on.